When Traditional Medicine Fails ... answers your questions on mold toxins and their impact on youth health, behavior and emotions.

- ☑ Is your child struggling with his or her health, behavior, mood, or schoolwork?
- ☑ Do you feel medications, counseling or tutoring are not hitting a "home run" with fixing your child's problem?
- ☑ If the EPA says 30% of all U.S. structures have significant indoor mold, and we know 10% of homes leak each year, what are the odds your child has dodged an indoor mold problem?
- ☑ Are you sure your family's allergy-like symptoms are just routine "allergies" or are you also feeling fogginess, fatigue or moodiness?
- ☑ If mold toxin illness training is absent from virtually ALL medical schools and residency programs, what are the odds that smart and sincere doctors will diagnose it?
- ☑ Biotoxins from hidden indoor mold can hurt your child in over 200 possible ways. How will your child's pediatrician diagnose these in a five-minute office visit?
- ☑ We will help YOU heal your child with our simple, powerful and cutting-edge options. We include clear legal pointers to beat the games of insurance companies, builders and school officials.
- ☑ Don't play Russian roulette with your child's (and your own) health. Read this book!

When Traditional Medicine Fails:

Your Guide to MOLD TOXINS

Revised 2nd Edition

Gary Rosen, Ph.D.
James Schaller, M.D.

Hope Academic Press

Published by: Hope Academic Press Tampa, Florida
Edited and formatted by Brad Moczik.

Printed in the United States of America

ISBN: 0-9773971-6-5

Forward

by James Schaller, M.D.

Take Back Your Children from Indoor Mold

I routinely treat children and adolescents who have problems with behavior and learning, and I treat over a hundred common causes for these youth problems. Want to be shocked? The most common cause for their problems is indoor mold contamination. This problem, often called Sick School Syndrome or Sick Building Syndrome (SBS), is caused by water leaks and excessive humidity inside a sealed building.

Until recently, few physicians had any understanding of SBS. Few understood that mold toxins from Sick Schools and Buildings can undermine child health, learning and behavior.

The recent EPA-funded study[1] *Guidance for Clinicians on the Recognition and Management of Health Effects Related to Mold Exposure and Moisture Indoors* has started to turn a few physicians around. The study advises medical clinicians to be on the lookout for neurological affects from indoor mold.

Now a few pediatricians and allergists are starting to recommend mold testing to confirm indoor mold exposure, followed by a "prescription" for mold remediation as part of a cure. But most physicians still don't get it.

Most have not read this important EPA-funded study and other recent research showing mold as a common cause of illness.

New breakthroughs in scientific techniques are quickly changing the face of medicine—including the field of mold-related illnesses. But most sincere physicians are just not able to keep up.

Fortunately, we can help. We are specialists in the field of mold toxins and their impact on human health. In this second edition of *When Traditional Medicine Fails*, we include critical new information to help you and your physician cure mold related ailments.

Mold DNA Profiling of Sick Buildings

Just a few years ago, no one had access to powerful DNA profiling technology, which became a household term during the O.J. Simpson case when it was used to profile human DNA. Now DNA profiling is used to characterize mold growth both in sick buildings and sick people. Its use and development was funded by the United States EPA.

New EPA research[2,3,4,5] shows that:

- ☑ 34 million Americans or 1 in 9 people have ongoing severe nasal and sinus infections or Chronic Rhinosinusitus (C.R.);
- ☑ C.R. is a direct result of molds that produce toxins growing in the sinuses of ill individuals, causing massive inflammation of the sinuses;
- ☑ The DNA profile of mold colonizing the sinuses of sick individuals **matches** the DNA profile of toxin-producing molds found in "sick" homes;
- ☑ The DNA profile of mold found in healthy homes was completely **different** from the mold found in C.R. patients' sinuses. Non-toxic molds were found in healthy homes;
- ☑ This U.S. study was repeated in the U.K. and had the same results.

Unfortunately for you and your loved ones, traditional medicine often does not keep up with the latest technology. Most physicians do not know about DNA profiling for mold or how to use it to help you.

In a similar fashion, new breakthroughs by numerous medical research groups in the United States and Europe show that many neurological symptoms are a direct result of "breathing" toxins produced by the same toxin-producing molds found in Sick Buildings.

In Chapter 3, we discuss the latest report published by the U.S. Surgeon General on recently declassified Army research revealing that mold neurotoxins have been used in biowarfare.

The research includes studies on human subjects showing that neurological disorders from exposures to mold biowarfare agents correlate with neurological disorders from Sick Buildings.

U.S. Army research also discusses toxin-binding treatments to cure neurotoxin exposure. These treatments are very much in line with the treatments developed by Ritchie Shoemaker, a prolific physician, and Kenneth Hudnell, an EPA scientist. Toxin-binding treatments are discussed further in Chapter 12.

We recommend that you review the 2004 publication by the National Academy of Science, *Damp Indoor Spaces*, starting with the section on Neurotoxic Affects of Mold on page 157.

Here is an excerpt:

> *Neurotoxic mycotoxins tend to fall into three general classes: tremor-genic toxins, paralytic toxins, and toxins that interfere with neurotransmitters or receptors either centrally or at the target organ.*
>
> *Many of the toxins are very potent and have immediate effects on animals exposed to a single dose by various routes.* (page 160)

While mold toxins cause dozens of common problems to the brain beyond these three basic categories, the quote confirms that indoor mold can cause much more than a *runny nose*.

Unlike typical bacterial and viral infections, mold toxins harm a very wide range of body functions and can make the diagnosis a bit tricky to the untrained eye.

What We Now Know About Mold and Neurotoxicity

Some people come to me (Schaller) after months or even years of traditional allergy testing, child psychiatry or pediatric drug treatments, yeast-free diets, gluten-free diets, fad diets for this and that, brain scans, numerous psychological and neurological tests, blood tests, and urine tests ... none of them helped!

Routinely, because of a lack of knowledge, sincere parents, teachers, schools, aunts, uncles, grandparents, clergy, pediatricians, and counselors will miss SBS as a cause for numerous youth troubles including both learning and behavioral problems. They simply do not know the impact that indoor mold can have on youth health. This book unravels the mysteries of mold biotoxin illness, and will guide you and your child to a path of recovery.

We now know ...

☑ **That the billions of dollars being spent on prescription drugs to treat illnesses from Sick Buildings NEVER WILL BE effective. Traditional drug therapies only treat the symptoms and do not cure. These make drug companies rich, but keep your child sick.**

☑ **When children suffer from multiple symptoms involving several organ groups, and when traditional medical testing does not find the problem, biotoxin exposure from indoor mold growth is often the source of the illness. While the symptoms can seem somewhat mysterious to the untrained, mold biotoxin illness can be treated successfully.**

Do You See Andrew's Problem?

Andrew transferred to a respected private school. At the beginning of the school year, he had trouble following directions and had an "ill mood" according to his strict teacher. His parents also noticed that Andrew seemed to be moodier. He was complaining that the classroom was "too loud" and he seemed to exaggerate physical contact with siblings and friends. His sleep was restless. Andrew wanted to have more time with his mother and to sleep in his parent's bed (even though he had stopped this behavior three years ago).

He was found to have both depressed alpha MSH, a critical hormone with over twenty functions, and increased blood inflammation (high MMP-9 and C3a). Plus, DNA studies showed that his genetic make-up included a vulnerability to mold toxins. Furthermore, his school had documented mold problems.

All these indicators strongly pointed toward mold toxins as the cause of illness.

After he was removed from the moldy school and given treatment for mold toxins, Andrew started getting better immediately. He was home schooled for 6 weeks and now is in a new school. Leaving the school certainly was an extreme solution and is not always needed. But after his mother tested two of the school's fan blades and the school's crusty, old AC filters, she found high levels of illness-promoting mold—not just the routine molds usually found indoors. She insisted on a new, mold-free school.

The parents spoke with their pediatrician and allergist about the mold sampling results along with the blood test findings from our lab. They also discussed Andrew's improvements. The pediatrician and allergist apparently had no real reply. These physicians had no idea what any of these tests meant. They admitted that they had neither read any of the latest research on the treatment of mold-related illnesses nor been trained in this type of illness.

But what is important is that Andrew is improving–his behavior is returning to normal. I just saw a picture of him, and he was clearly happy in the photo. Good for him and his loving sacrificial parents!

Behavior and Learning Challenges

In the outdoors, there are tens of thousands of competing species of mold. Living outdoors is tough for molds. Most can barely survive outdoors with the thousands of competitors, UV radiation, rain, temperature fluctuations, and wind. A home or school with a moist indoors offers molds a much easier life. And as a result, when living indoors, their ability to make biotoxins, which they use to kill other molds and bacteria, is greatly enhanced.

Low levels of indoor mold growth can adversely affect sensitive children.

Today's common household materials such as wallboard, carpet and wood—along with today's tighter, more energy-efficient buildings that keep out fresh, outside air—are what most toxin-producing molds thrive on. Just add water.

After two to three days, a wet indoor setting can start producing mold. Once the mold starts, it will continue to grow with only humidity. Mold spreads fast, and the biotoxins they produce to kill other molds and bacteria can make people ill. Initially, most people are entirely clueless that they are being affected. Sickness can come on gradually as mold biotoxins pass from cell to cell with great ease—altering DNA and hurting children and their parents.

Unlike typical viral or bacterial infections, mold toxins can be active throughout virtually the entire body and can cause a diverse array of child health problems. That is why they can be hard to diagnose. While mold-related health problems affect people of all ages and both sexes, research shows that children are particularly vulnerable. Common symptoms include:

- ✓ Poor attention span
- ✓ Limited ability to focus
- ✓ Irritability
- ✓ Headaches
- ✓ Mood swings
- ✓ Disobedience
- ✓ Homework difficulty
- ✓ Difficulty in learning
- ✓ Anxiety
- ✓ Agitation
- ✓ Excess aggression
- ✓ Difficulty relating to peers

Do you think mold problems are rare? The EPA reports that 30% of all U.S. structures have indoor mold. And how often do you hear of a roof leak in a home or a school? I routinely hear of homes or offices having a “small leak” or a “little water in the basement.” People calmly mention an annoying little leak, and talk about having a plumber come “in a few days.” They mention this “leak” casually. But indoor mold is not a casual topic. Every year one in ten homes has an indoor leak.

And every year, schools turn off their air conditioning during August, inadvertently creating a highly humid and stale indoor environment that is perfect for mold growth. Hidden mold growth in water-damaged schools and in homes is a major child issue.

With these facts in mind, I am delighted to introduce *When Traditional Medicine Fails: Your Guide to Mold Toxins* ... a new weapon to protect the children you love.

In *When Traditional Medicine Fails*, we provide fresh insight into the four critical areas concerning mold toxin exposure:

Diagnosis: We fully and clearly explain mold toxin symptoms and explain which children are most likely to become ill from mold. Specifically, we offer material and cases showing how mold toxins affect behavior, insight, mood, concentration, memory, personality, and achievement. You won’t find this material anywhere else.

Mold Clean-Up: We show you the proper way to remove mold and mold toxins from both homes and schools. Curing your child includes carefully removing mold and toxins without further contaminating the building. We explain how you can make your home “as good as new.”

Ongoing Healthy Environment: Humidity control and air filtration are powerful tools to continually eliminate from indoor air even trace amounts of not only mold spores and their toxins, but also bacteria, viruses, and other pollutants. We explain in detail what you need to know to provide a healthy indoor environment for your children and entire family.

Treatment Options: We offer many specific ways to restore your child to full health, including the use of mold toxin binders to cure mold toxin exposure before it seriously alters your child’s body chemistry. You will be given many tools and options to obtain the best treatment for your child.

I am deeply honored to co-author this expanded and fully revised version with Dr. Rosen. I think you will find it a mix of clear writing, cutting-edge medicine, and practical advice on how to fix mold-related problems.

We feel this short book is the simplest and fastest way to reclaim your child's life from environmental illness caused by indoor mold growth.

James Schaller, M.D., M.A.R., C.M.R., C.M.I.
Director, Professional Medical Services of Naples

www.usmoldphysician.com
Co-author of *Mold Warriors: Fighting America's Hidden Health Threat*

Author of *Mold Illness Made Simple*

The next few pages depict several sample images of common toxin-producing molds, along with descriptions of just some of their adverse effects on human health.

PENICILLIUM sp.

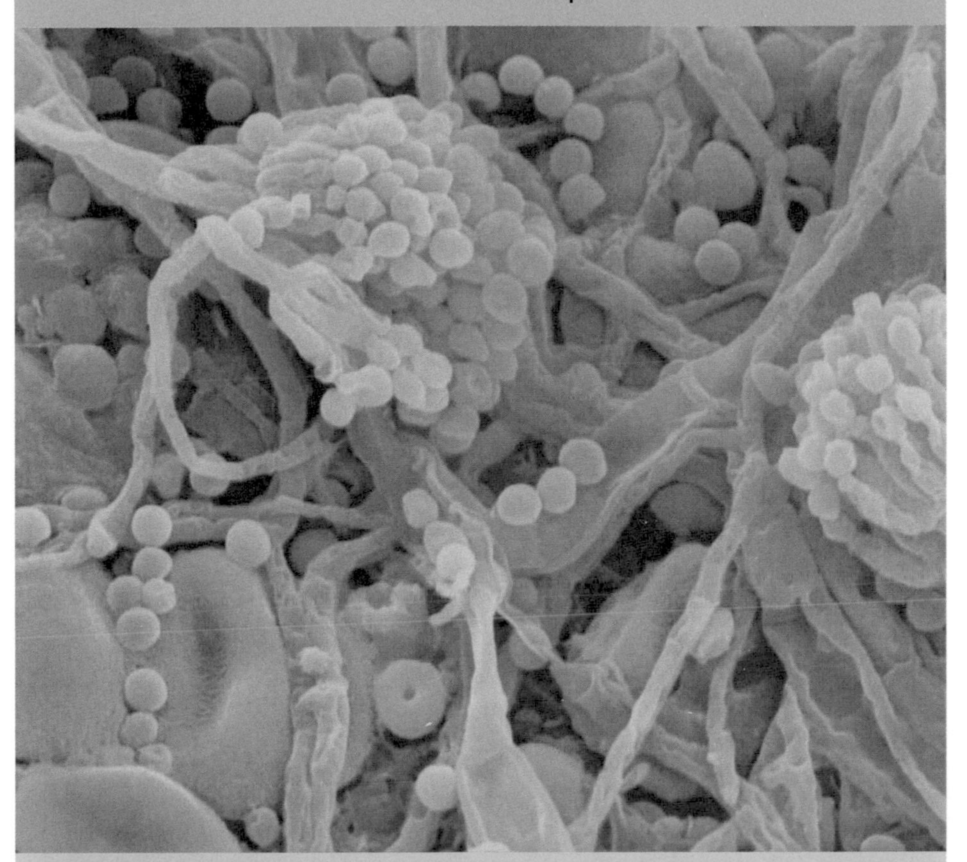

ALLERGENICITY:	Allergenic.
MYCOTOXINS PRODUCED:	Various toxins by different species: Anacine, Arisugacins A&B, Auranthine(sclerotigenin), Aurantiamine, Belfedrin A, Botryodiplodin, Brevianamid A, Chaetoglobosin A, B&C, Chlororugulovasines A&B, Chrysogine, Citromycetin, Citreoisocoumarinol, Citreoviridin, Citrinin, Communensins A&B, Compactin, Curvularin, Cyanein, Cyclochlorotine, Cyclopenin, Cyclopenol, Cyclopiazonic acid, Cytostipin, etc. Complete list available at reference below.
HUMAN PATHOGENICITY:	Bronchopulmonary, nail, (sub)cutaneous, ear infections; systemic disease; osteomyelitis; endophthalmitis; keratitis; esophagitis; pericarditis; endocarditis. Effects found mostly in immunocompromised patients.
REFERENCE:	http://www.ttuhsc.edu/SOM/Microbiology/mainweb/aiaq/Glossary.html

ASPERGILLUS ochraceous

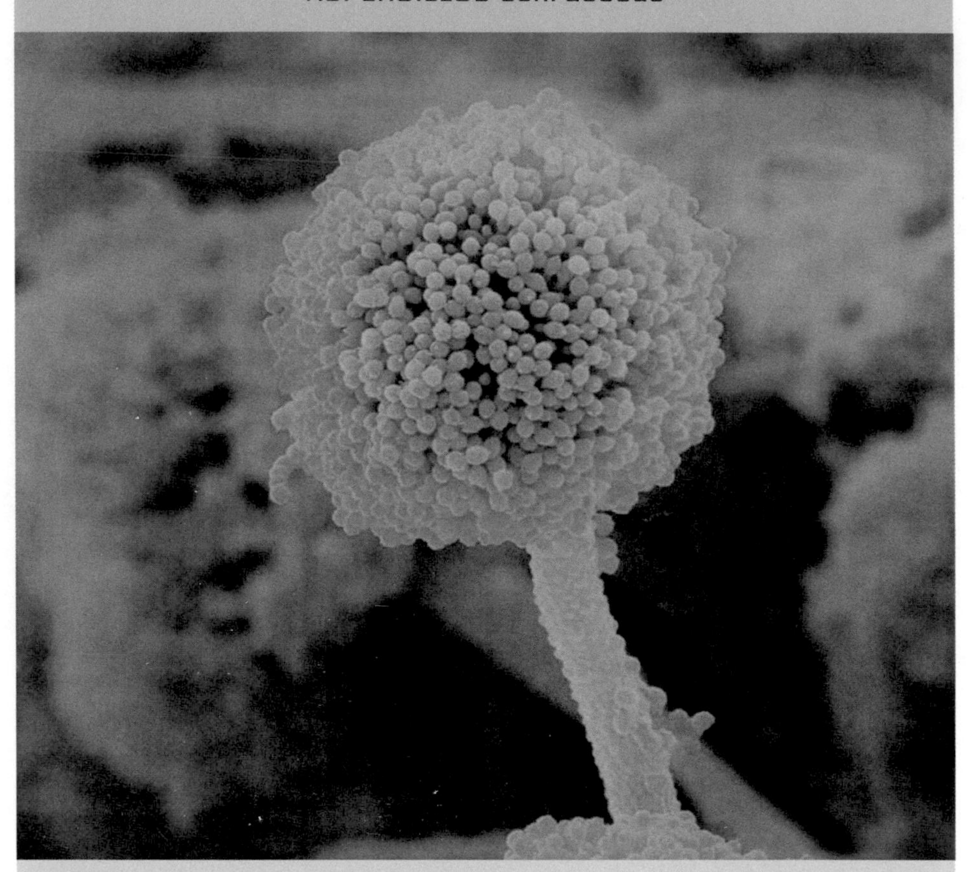

ALLERGENICITY:	Allergenic.
MYCOTOXINS PRODUCED:	Ochratoxin, Penicillic acid.
HUMAN PATHOGENICITY:	Antromycosis; mycotoxin-induced tubulonephritis; chronic interstitial nephropathy.
REFERENCE:	http://www.ttuhsc.edu/SOM/Microbiology/mainweb/aiaq/Glossary.html

STACHYBOTRYS sp.

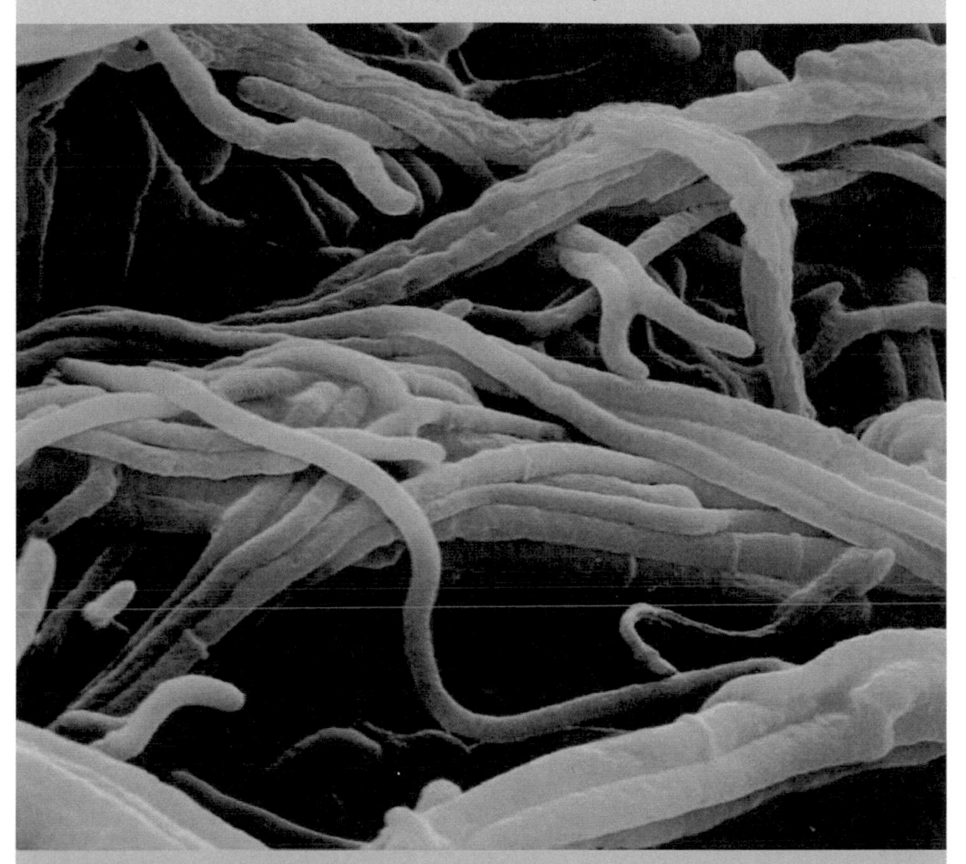

ALLERGENICITY:	Can be allergenic.
MYCOTOXINS PRODUCED:	3-Acetyl-deoxynivalenol , Atranones A-G, Cyclosporins, Diacetoxyscirpenol, Deoxynivalenol or Vomitoxin, Epoxytrichothecene, Isosatratoxins F, G & H, Phenylspirodrimanes, Roridins A, E, Satratoxins F, G & H, Stachylysin, Trichoverrols A, B, Verrucarins A,J, Verrucarol (T-2-tetraol).
HUMAN PATHOGENICITY:	Mycotoxin-caused pulmonary hemorrhage/hemosiderosis in infants; dermatitis; cough; rhinitis; itching or burning sensation in mouth, throat, nasal passages, and eyes.
REFERENCE:	http://www.ttuhsc.edu/SOM/Microbiology/mainweb/aiaq/Glossary.html

ASPERGILLUS clavatus

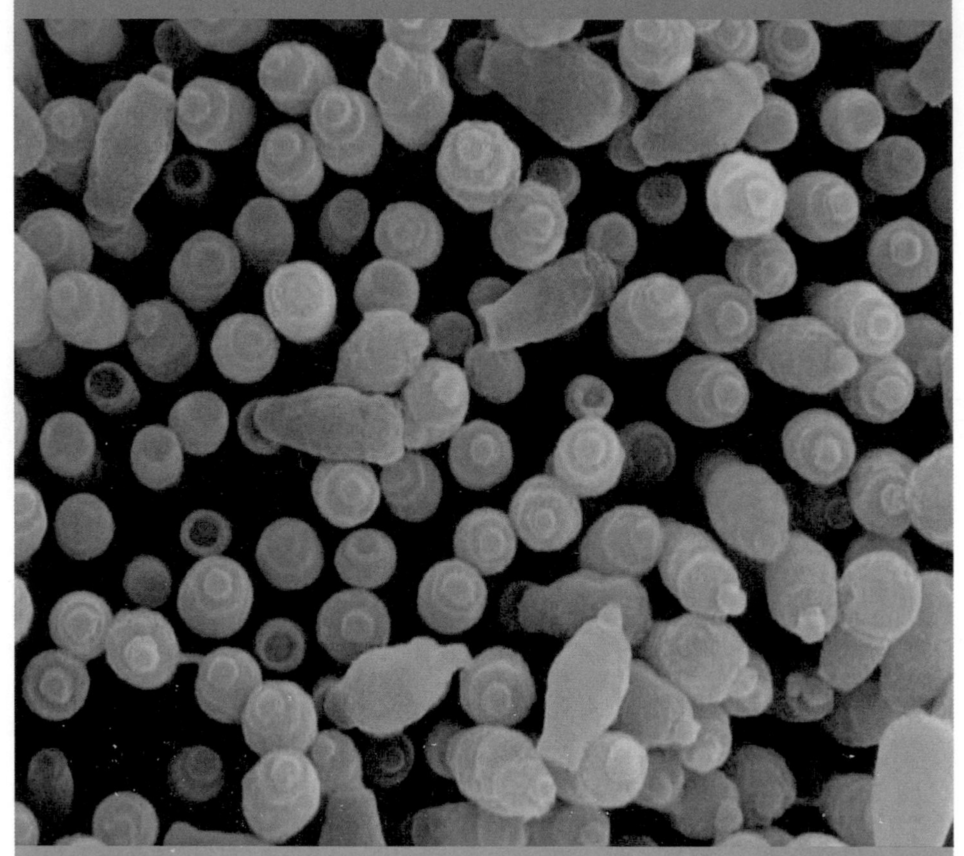

ALLERGENICITY:	Allergenic.
MYCOTOXINS PRODUCED:	Ascladiol, Brefeldin A, Cytochalasin E, Ribotoxins, Patulin, Triptoquivalins.
HUMAN PATHOGENICITY:	Agent of allergic aspergillosis, pulmonary infection, and endocarditis.
REFERENCE:	http://www.ttuhsc.edu/SOM/Microbiology/mainweb/aiaq/Glossary.html

ASPERGILLUS niger

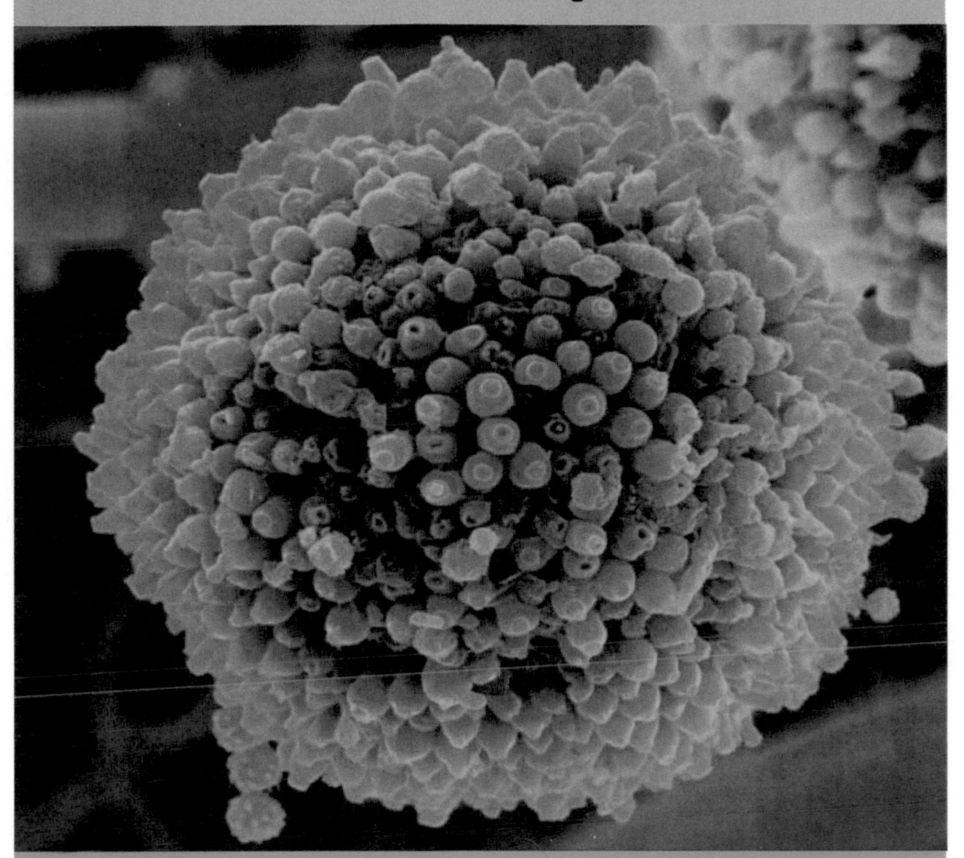

ALLERGENICITY:	Allergenic.
MYCOTOXINS PRODUCED:	Malformins B&C, Naphtho-gamma-pyrones, Ochratoxin A, Oxalic acid.
HUMAN PATHOGENICITY:	Etiologic agent of otomycosis; "Swimmer's ear;" onychomycosis; can cause bronchopulmonary, pulmonary, nasosinus aspergillosis; pneumonia; eye infections; invasive lung, heart and other disease.
REFERENCE:	http://www.ttuhsc.edu/SOM/Microbiology/mainweb/aiaq/Glossary.html

SCOPULARIOPSIS sp.

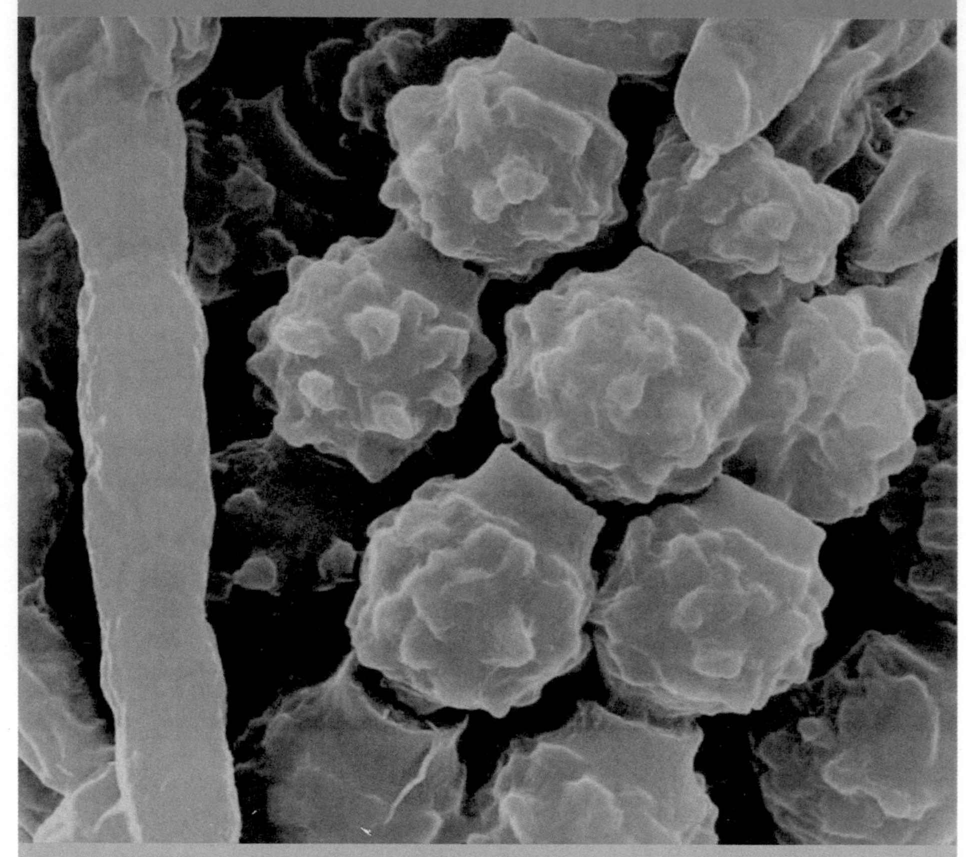

ALLERGENICITY:	Allergenic.
MYCOTOXINS PRODUCED:	Unknown.
HUMAN PATHOGENICITY:	Onychomycosis; pulmonary mycosis; invasive human infections; sub-cutaneous infections, keratitis, endophthalmitis, mycetoma; cerebral infections.
REFERENCE:	http://www.ttuhsc.edu/SOM/Microbiology/mainweb/aiaq/Glossary.html

FUSARIUM sp.

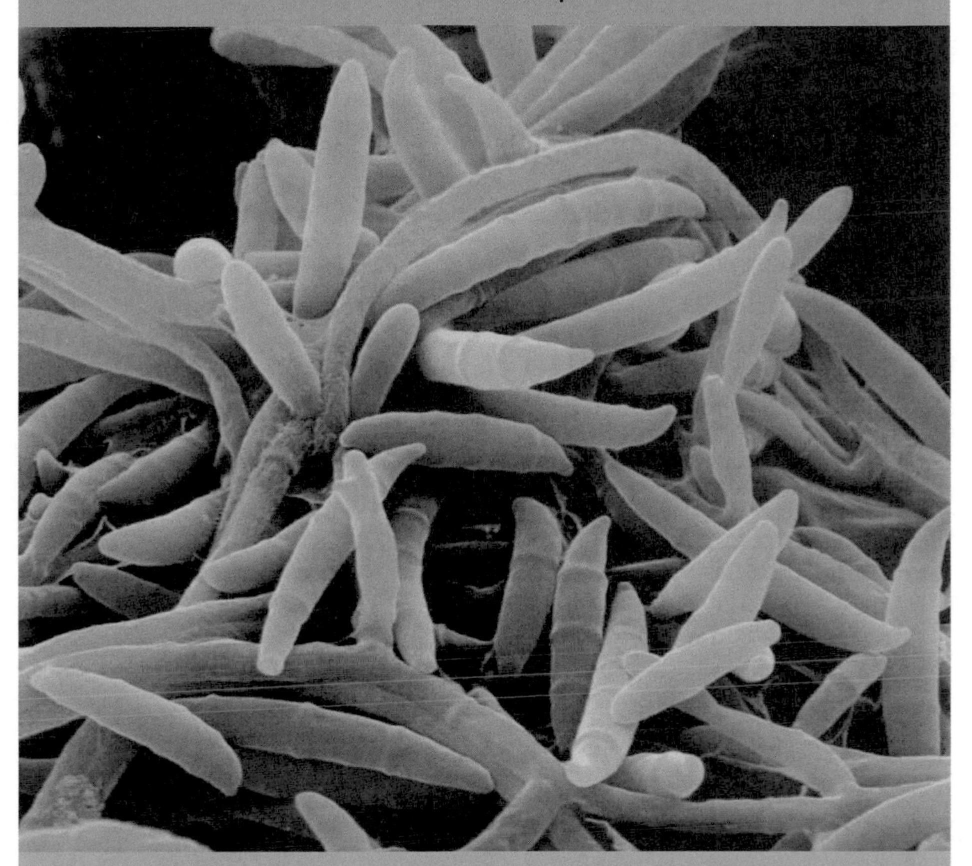

ALLERGENICITY:	Allergenic.
MYCOTOXINS PRODUCED:	Acetoxyscirpenol, Acetoxyscirpentriol, Acetyldeoxynivalenol, 3-Acetyl-neosolaniol, 15-Acetyl-nivalenol, 3-Acetyl-HT-2 toxin, Acetyl-T-2-tetraol, Acetyl-T-2 toxin, Acuminatopyrone, Antibiotic Y, Apotrichothecenes, Beauvericin, Butenolide, Calonectrin, Chlamydospordiol, Chlamydosporol, Culmorin, Deacylcalonectrin, Deoxyfusapyrone, Deoxynivalenol (Vomitoxin), Diacetyl-nivalenol, Diacetoxyscirpenol, etc. Complete list available at reference below.
HUMAN PATHOGENICITY:	Causes eye, (sub)cutaneous, nail, pulmonary, and heart infections; mycetomas; arthritis; peritonitis; cerebral, disseminated, or systemic opportunistic infections in immunocompromised patients.
REFERENCE:	http://www.ttuhsc.edu/SOM/Microbiology/mainweb/aiaq/Glossary.html

DISCLAIMER

The products and the claims made about specific products on or through this book have not been evaluated by the United States Food and Drug Administration and are not approved to diagnose, treat, cure, or prevent disease. The information provided in this book is for informational purposes only and is not intended as a substitute for advice from your physician or other health care professional. Any information in this book is not intended to replace any information contained on or in any product label or packaging. You should not use the information in this book for diagnosis or treatment of any health problem, or for prescription of any medication or other treatment. You should consult with a health care professional: before starting any diet, exercise or supplementation program; before taking any medication; or if you have, or suspect you might have, a health problem.

Introduction

Do you know what some species of spiders, snakes, scorpions, bees, and ticks have in common with mold and mushrooms? They make biotoxin poisons. Biotoxins are toxins made by living organisms. The table below lists just a few of the species that produce biotoxins along with the names of the toxins.

Name of Toxin	Source	Name of Toxin	Source
Agitoxin	Scorpion	**Ergot Alkaloids**	**Aspergillus Mold**
Alpha-bungarotoxin	Krait (snake)	Grammotoxin SIA	Rose Tarantula
Anatoxin	Algae	Holocyclotoxin	Paralysis Tick
Apamin	Honey Bee	Kaliotoxin	Scorpion
Batrachotoxin	Arrow Frog	Latrotoxin	Black Widow Spider
Botulinum toxin	Bacteria	**LSD**	**Toxic Fungi**
Brevetoxin	Red Tide	Maculotoxin	Blue-Ringed Octopus
Cobrotoxin	Cobra Snake	**Ochratoxin**	**Penicillium Mold**
Conotoxin	Marine Snail	Philanthotoxin	Predaceous Wasp
Crotoxin	Rattlesnake	SNX-482	African Tarantula
Erabutoxin	Sea Snake	**Tricothecene**	**Stachybotrys Mold**

Biotoxins are produced as powerful defensive or offensive chemicals, used to crowd out or capture prey. In the case of mold, biotoxins are meant to kill bacteria, other molds and various mites. But just like biotoxins from poisonous snakes and scorpions, mold-produced biotoxins can definitely hurt humans.

So, what happens to children in a mold-contaminated school or moldy home filled with biotoxins? How do mold biotoxins affect them? The answer is ... it depends. It depends on the amount of exposure and how well a particular child can remove biotoxins from their body—a function that is highly variable from child to child.

When a bee stings you, you know what is making you sick. But with slow-acting mold biotoxin exposure from a Sick Building, it is not so easy to tell exactly what is causing the illness.

Indoor mold growth is a problem that affects millions of children and adults. Chronically breathing mold toxins over extended periods of time can cause subtle and diverse symptoms. As the duration and amount of exposure increase, serious child or adult emotional and behavior problems can occur. Because the biotoxins are flowing through the blood stream for extended periods of time, they can target most of the organs in the body—including the brain. Resulting symptoms can affect virtually all body organs and systems. However ...

> Did you know?
>
> **Approximately 1 in 4 children does not remove mold biotoxins well and will be affected by even moderately elevated levels of indoor mold growth.**

The amazing thing about mold toxin exposure is that it can often be quickly and easily cured when:

☑ Properly diagnosed;

☑ Some select interventions are used;

☑ And further toxin exposure is eliminated or minimized.

This book started out about Johnny. He lives next door. He had been cured of serious learning troubles along with many physical ailments, seemingly miraculously, after only one visit to Dr. Ritchie Shoemaker and aggressive treatment with Cholestyramine (CSM), a mold toxin binder.

The CSM toxin binder works naturally by helping the body more efficiently eliminate toxins.

Millions of Johnnys

Then I met Dr. James Schaller, a well-respected Florida physician and child psychiatrist, who also treats patients nationwide for biotoxin exposure. Through discussions with Dr. Schaller, it became apparent to me that Johnny's biotoxin-related environmental illness is being played out with millions of children all over the country.

Until Johnny was in the seventh grade, his reading ability was normal. Over the next several years, his reading and math skills remained stuck at a seventh-grade level. What happened?

The library had a leaky roof. We now know that toxic mold contaminated the entire library. The teachers and children just thought the library was "a little musty." But that smell was from living mold that was actively producing toxins! So Johnny sat in the library during study hall inhaling toxins. These caused him to develop neurological symptoms that affected his concentration and overall mental ability. He was diagnosed with Attention Deficit Disorder (ADD) and his reading and math grades fell.

After several years of exposure, his subtle learning limitations became severe. He then left school due to overwhelming academic problems. At the same time, he had headaches, sinus infections, low energy, stomach aches, reduced coordination, and body rashes.

He tested negative for every kind of allergy. He had numerous courses of antibiotics for sinus infections; he had a brain scan; he had his lungs X-rayed. He tested negative for Lyme, even from the elite tick lab, IGeneX. He even went to a psychologist. Maybe he just could not cope with school stress and all the problems were psychosomatic?

Doctors were baffled. No one had any idea what would cause these problems much less how to treat them. Why would an excellent student like Johnny suddenly develop ADD in the *seventh grade*? Kids do not develop ADD in middle school. And what about his other symptoms? What no one knew at the time was that all of his problems were typical of Sick School Syndrome.

Biotoxins in the Air our Children Breath

While the majority of children in Johnny's school showed no symptoms of toxic mold exposure, medical tests showed that Johnny's genetics cause him to take longer to clear toxins from his body than most other kids. If he is in a sick school or home, toxins will build up in his body and Johnny will get sick. In all other respects, he is like other healthy kids. He was rarely ill before the library exposure.

Johnny's experience and symptoms are not unique. We know schools are notoriously under-funded and that water damage and the resulting mold growth is common. ACs are often turned off to save money, allowing humidity to climb to mold-producing levels. In humid or water-damaged schools, illness from hidden toxic mold is often the single biggest cause of childhood medical, emotional, behavioral, and learning disorders.

- ☑ The problems start with water or excess indoor humidity from leaky roofs, faulty AC systems or AC systems turned off for days to "save money." Any of these can give rise to indoor mold growth.
- ☑ The problems expand as school officials deny the latest scientific evidence that shows common *Penicillium* and *Aspergillus* molds, routinely growing in water-damaged buildings, produce harmful toxins. When our kids inhale these toxins daily, some can become emotionally and physically troubled.
- ☑ The medical problems reach epidemic proportions when school officials ignore laws that require classrooms to be ventilated with clean outside air that "washes away" mold toxins and other indoor-air pollutants. To save on heating and air conditioning costs, windows and vents remain closed and indoor air is recycled. Kids remain bottled up in classrooms with contaminated air as hidden mold growing in water-damaged walls, ceilings and air ducts releases toxins.

Nationally, millions of children need to have complex educational plans, attend special schools, or stay at home. Many of these children are sick from mold-related illnesses that are often labeled as emotional or behavioral problems and learning disorders.

These disorders often decrease and or are eliminated when the students no longer attend water-damaged schools. But no one seems to understand why. School officials and physicians miss the obvious cause: illness from toxins in the sick school they attended.

School officials, parents, and the public in general need to face some clear facts:

- ☑ Humidity in excess of 65% in a school, home or office will foster mold growth and biotoxin production. This scenario is very common and routinely missed.
- ☑ Symptoms from water-damaged schools go far beyond asthma, nasal allergies or a runny nose.
- ☑ You do not need to be diagnosed with a mold allergy to become sick from mold toxins. Mold toxin poisoning has nothing to do with allergic reactions to mold.
- ☑ Mold-contaminated schools or homes often cause neurological and psychiatric problems in children as well as teachers and parents.
- ☑ Psychiatric problems can include mild or severe anxiety, irritability, boredom, agitation, anger, decreased focusing ability, obsession, depression, panic attacks, impulsivity, attention troubles, fighting, and eccentric behavior.
- ☑ Neurological and medical disorders can include fatigue, muscle aches, headaches, sinus congestion, and asthma. These disorders do not fully respond to normal treatments. In addition, there can be memory loss, lack of concentration, metallic taste, sensitivity to bright light, and subtle vision abnormalities.

Despite clear information on the adverse health affects from mold toxins, including data from EPA studies, school officials continue to ignore the hazards of indoor mold growth ... including the need to be on the lookout for neurological disorders from indoor mold. Schools continue to deny, trivialize and cover up toxic mold problems in their sick schools. But by covering up the problems, the proper diagnosis is not made, sick students are not treated, and the problems become much bigger. In the private sector, facilities managers are put in jail for covering up hazardous environments. But in schools, the cover-ups continue even in light of government research about the many neurotoxins from mold found in water-damaged buildings.

School officials cling to an old pathetic defense: "Since not every child is sick, the cause of illness must lie outside the school."

But we have known for decades that drugs and poisons affect everyone at a *different* dose. And we now know that approximately 1 out of 4 children are genetically vulnerable to mold. Their bodies cannot effectively remove mold toxins.

Medical Diagnosis

What is necessary for the diagnosis of Sick Building Syndrome due to indoor mold toxin exposure is:

- ☑ Exposure to a school or home with visible or musty smelling indoor mold.
- ☑ Chronic symptoms that fail routine treatment.
- ☑ The presence of mold-specific blood results easily seen in certain lab tests.
- ☑ Finally, most children feel better when they are away from a moldy home or school. But if a child has been exposed to mold toxins too long or too intensely, they may not improve without treatment even when away from the problem building.

Mold toxins are usually misdiagnosed and treated with extensive antibiotics, antihistamines, steroids, and a wide range of psychiatric medications—often making matters worse.

Just as we now know that many chronic sinus infections are from mold and not bacteria, many chronic illnesses, as well as behavior and learning struggles, are from homes or schools with mold contamination.

Our Goal and Hope

We are writing to help you and your child find a correct diagnosis and the corresponding solutions.

When Traditional Medicine Fails unravels the mysteries of toxic mold related illnesses. We clearly and concisely answer your questions:

- ☑ How do I know if mold toxins are the cause of my child's problems? What are the exact symptoms of Sick Building Syndrome?
- ☑ What about adults? Can mold toxin exposure cause such diverse symptoms as headaches, poor concentration, sleep problems, and even sexual dysfunction in adults?
- ☑ What common molds release harmful chemicals?
- ☑ What are the health treatment options? Are over-the-counter solutions available? If so, how do they compare to prescription medications?
- ☑ Do I really need to spend thousands on mold testing and/or mold remediation? How do I choose a good mold tester or mold remediator? What can I do myself?
- ☑ Are there any simple solutions to reduce my child's exposure levels in a mold-contaminated home or school?
- ☑ My doctor does not know much about mold toxins and treatments. What treatment options can I suggest to my doctor?

In short, *When Traditional Medicine Fails* is your guide to mold toxins: what they are; how they can alter your child's behavior and learning; and how to get rid of them and reclaim your child's health, learning and behavior.

CHAPTER 1

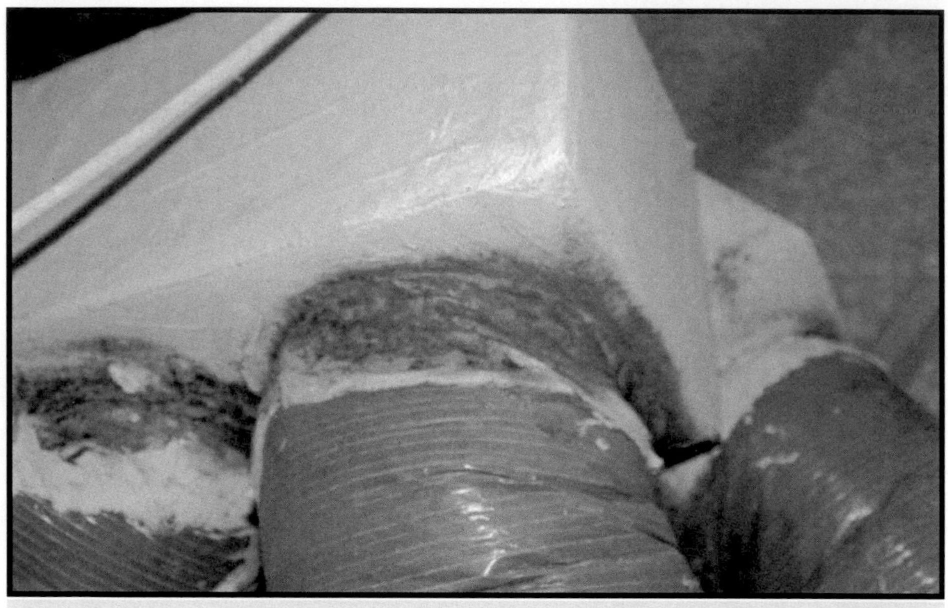

A duct leak in the attic caused this mold growth. The residents inside were getting sick because the hatch to the attic did not close well. If the house is properly sealed from the attic, moderate mold growth in the attic usually will not make people inside the home sick.

Everyday Observations of Mold-Related Problems in Students, School Staff & Parents

Mold toxins can affect sensitive children and adults in numerous ways. These toxins impact the brain directly and increase many types of inflammation chemicals. Mold toxins also alter many hormone levels. All of these anomalies are usually missed by routine medical exams unless mold toxin-related symptoms are specifically investigated. Further, mold toxins can cause subtle but serious personality changes. Do any of the people in the following case studies seem like you, your child, or your child's teacher?

Decreased Learning Capacity

Ricky has had a reading disability for the last five years. Clearly, when he started at his middle school this past September, his ability to learn dropped immensely. Previously, he was able to get Bs, but now he was failing English. Only after reading a paragraph repeatedly could he recall the general point.

Ricky's father took swab samples from the areas that he suspected might be mold. They came back positive for toxic mold. A few of the problem areas also came back showing toxin-making bacteria called "gram-negative bacilli." These "bacilli" or hot dog shaped bacteria have toxins on their outer coating and can reduce the educational ability of youth who are in contact with them.

The school would not accept the results, partly because their "expert" had tested the school earlier and had reported it was fine. Ricky was home schooled for the rest of the year. After three months away from the moldy school, Ricky started to improve academically. Legal action is still pending.

Impulsivity

"I think it is sixty four!" Anthony yelled out. His teacher forced a small smile. She was tired of his calling out even though he meant well. He did the same thing with his friends and family. He was not this way a year ago, and his mother had no idea what caused this change.

Anthony had a humidifier in his room during the winter, when his home was below 40% humidity and the low humidity would cause his skin to crack—especially if he took hot showers.

His home was inspected for mold. The worst source was the humidifier in his room, filled with thousands of mold colonies and millions of toxic bacteria, which thrive in dirty water.

Dead Creativity

Julie was a good student and enjoyed both music and pencil drawing. Yet for two years she left her flute and sketch pad sitting in her bedroom drawer. After school she seemed to be worn, as if she just finished an aggressive work-out.

Blood testing showed her VEGF and MSH labs were very low. The low levels reduced her energy and lowered her mood and enjoyment.

Her parents swore there was no mold in their home. But an infrared thermographic camera found three moisture sources in her walls. Upon further investigation, mold was found. The contaminated drywall was removed, some carpet was thrown out, and the contaminated areas were HEPA vacuumed.

It took a while, but eventually Julie's VEGF and MSH returned to normal. She is back playing her flute and drawing.

The Obvious Comes Slowly

A father and son had trouble from toxic mold exposure but neither knew it. The sixteen-year-old son was in a residential treatment facility that refused Dr. Schaller's input. After Michael was discharged, we found he had serious mold toxins in his Texas home. He showed massive inflammation in his body from many important lab tests, including a MMP-9. Generally, we like to see MMP-9 far under 250 and he had an 855! His brain was being bathed in inflammatory "gasoline" that hindered him mentally and physically.

We removed the four sources of mold in his home and "mopped up" the mold toxins in his body with the toxin-binding agent, Cholestyramine. In five months he was free of all ailments. He now has an A- average and is more sociable. Finally, after his home was remediated and tested to be free of indoor mold growth, and after our medical treatments, he yelled in amazement, "This is freaked out! After all those years of psychiatric medications and therapists, it all ended up being these environmental things and not me. This is amazing!"

The father had similar troubles, but refused to believe he was being affected by the same mold biotoxins that had been poisoning his son. Finally, after two full years of nagging, the father took my suggested lab tests, which showed massive mold biotoxin damage to his body including:

- ☑ Antibodies against the fat surrounding his nerves.
- ☑ Hormone changes resulting in high estrogen and low testosterone. This pattern may promote prostate cancer.

☑ A weak immune system including low natural killer cells—the ones that kill cancer every day.

☑ A significantly elevated risk of blood clotting.

He is getting better slowly, and now has better insight. But, the insight came only after the lab findings hit him in the face.

Common Frontal Lobe Signs of Mold Illness

Indoor mold decreases insight because of its impact on the front part of your brain, the "frontal lobe."

When we mention frontal lobe signs, we are referring to the detrimental effects mold has on the frontal lobe and its numerous functions. Think of this part of the brain as the top of a pyramid. And if a layer of bricks is out of place, the top of the pyramid will be "off." Similarly, if brain tissue is irritated or inflamed below the frontal lobe, it will impair the normal functions controlled by the frontal lobe.

This is why some psychiatrists, who are trained to detect subtle changes in brain chemistry, can be the first to notice mold-related illnesses. Similarly, parents generally are very tuned into their children and notice small behavioral, mood or personality changes that others might not notice. Parents' gut instincts are often right and can help speed a child to a diagnosis of mold toxin exposure.

Look over the list and illustration cases below. Do you see any of these frontal lobe signs in your child, yourself or school staff? Are any of these changes new and associated with exposure to water damage and/or a moldy smelling home or school?

- Moodiness and irritability
- Rigidity
- Impulsivity
- Poor insight
- New distractibility
- Trouble finishing a task

- Acting eccentrically or impulsively with money, drinking, drugs, sex, unwanted pregnancy or speech content
- Decreased speech speed and smoothness
- Decreased coordination
- Stress with transitions or change
- Routine lateness
- Empathic deficits
- New immature silliness
- Social deficits—making others uncomfortable
- Poor boundary awareness
- New aggressiveness
- Increased dependence in a child or adult

"Flaky"

Jennifer is called "flaky" because she is regularly distracted. She was not that way until she moved to Long Island at the age of seventeen. During the summer when she lives in another home, she is much less distracted. The basement in her primary home was found to have three species of toxic mold. Lab tests showed she had a low MSH level, which most likely was as a result of exposure to mold toxins.

"I Can't Get Things Done Any More"

Michele was a solid B student. After transferring into her new school, she started having trouble completing her homework. She could not go from A—Z and complete an assignment. Her mother feared she had gotten in with the "wrong crowd," and was concerned at Michele's red eyes and slowed thinking. Michele blamed her lower performance on her new teachers. She laughed at suspicions of drug use.

During a medical examination in my office, she challenged me to give her a drug test. I did. She handed the negative urine and blood results to her mother proudly.

Eventually, her mother learned from other parents and a few teachers that mold problems were suspected in the school. When I could not find another cause for Michele's symptoms—and her lab tests pointed toward mold—I suggested taking a few air samples at the school. A teacher confidentially handled the testing, which came back positive. The administration refused to consider the results, and so Michele transferred reluctantly to another school and is finally doing very well.

Ignorant Rigidity & Protectiveness

Mold victims can have trouble with new ideas. Learning new educational material requires a properly functioning brain. Those with mold-induced brain fog often feel uncomfortable and overwhelmed when dealing with new information.

Sometimes this shows up in reactions to my medical advice. I suggest patients get their home or school tested and, suddenly, "all knowing" relatives or friends offer their contrary opinion. Many of these naysayers live in their own moldy homes. Despite the fact that the ill children have seen five to forty previous doctors—with no success—ignorant relatives, friends and pseudosages try to save them *from me.*

I hate to say it, but sometimes the silly "sage" is a father who becomes annoyed at the mere mention of mold. When he thinks of mold he thinks of beer, old bread or the stuff in the forest. Commonly, if mold is in the father's home, the father is functioning far below his abilities, since he is breathing the toxins that the child is breathing. Even if he is very smart, his insight and other frontal lobe functions can be deficient.

Sometimes a spouse or a housemate sees a negative personality change in someone before that person can see it in himself. The wife sees her husband as too irritable and tired, while the husband sees his wife as snappy and foggy.

Narcissism or Profound Self-Centered Thinking

Alice is in high school and complains regularly. In a group session, she takes over conversations so she can talk about herself. When you talk with her, you sense she is not listening to you or connecting with you as a living person—you could just as easily be a stool. Her bed headboard was found to have *Aspergillus* and *Penicillium* molds at very high levels. So as she sleeps she breathes in toxic mold substances. Her labs showed depressed MSH and increased blood inflammation.

After thoroughly cleaning her bedroom, fixing the moisture problem in her attic that caused the mold growth, and treating her body with toxin-binding Cholestyramine, her personality started returning to normal. Her ability to care for and connect with others is clearly improved, and her lab results are normalizing.

Eccentric Personalities

Michael is "weird." His old friends noticed he was becoming weird when he was fourteen. Suddenly, all he would talk about was animals, guns and money. His mother brought him in for testing. His mold lab results were positive and he was also positive for Lyme and Bartonella—three conditions which impact the brain. His father said he was "just fine." Michael dropped out of school and now works for his father.

Organization Extremes

Joe has always liked order. Yet two years ago, after he transferred into a Votech center, his parent's noticed he was unsettled with even slight "disorder." He became annoyed if someone moved his CDs or his clothes had a wrinkle. His Votech center turned out to be positive for mold.

EPA Definition of Mycotoxins (1994)

Another class of agents that may cause disease related to indoor airborne exposure is the mycotoxins. These agents are fungal metabolites that have toxic effects ranging from short-term irritation to immuno-suppression and cancer. Virtually all the information related to diseases caused by mycotoxins concerns ingestion of contaminated food. However, mycotoxins are contained in some kinds of fungus spores, and these can enter the body through the respiratory tract. At least one case of neurotoxic symptoms possibly related to airborne mycotoxin exposure in a heavily contaminated environment has been reported. Skin is another potential route of exposure to mycotoxins. Toxins of several fungi have caused cases of severe dermatosis. In view of the serious nature of the toxic effects reported for mycotoxins, exposure to mycotoxin-producing agents should be minimized. *Indoor Air Pollution: An Introduction for Health Professionals*, U.S. Government Printing Office Publication No. 1994-523-217/81322, 1994 [EPA 402-R-94-007, 1994] http://www.epa.gov/iaq/pubs/hpguide.html#mycotoxins

CHAPTER 2

To be diagnosed with ADHD, a child must have a number of symptoms for six months, including frequent failure to pay attention during schoolwork or play, frequent mistakes due to inattention to schoolwork, frequent failure to listen when spoken to directly, forgetfullness, and failure to follow up on chores.

The Centers for Disease Control conservatively estimate that health care costs associated with ADHD are about $3.3 billion annually.

Is part of this increase in ADHD-like symptoms due to mold in schools? You bet!

EPA Scientist Discovers Cure

Once we understand that mold biotoxins can damage the body and nervous system and are common in water-damaged schools, homes and offices, we can start asking a few hard questions. For instance, since watchdog agencies like the Environmental Protection Agency (EPA) recognize that indoor mold growth can make you sick, why isn't the government doing more about it? Further, why isn't the government involved with mold toxin treatment when one of their own scientists helped prove that the toxin binder, Cholestyramine, helps remove biotoxins like those made by indoor mold?

Who Monitors Schools for Mold Toxins?

The EPA's mission is "to protect human health and to safeguard the air, water, and land upon which life depends." They have a highly educated staff of 9,000 that include engineers and scientists. So what are they doing to fix sick schools?

Almost nothing. While EPA scientists can study toxic mold, it turns out the EPA's authority suddenly stops at the schoolhouse doors. The agency is a watchdog only over *outdoor* pollutants; it cannot regulate inside ones.

What about OSHA, the Occupational Safety and Health Administration? OSHA's mission is to "save lives, prevent injuries and protect the health of America's workers." That means employers and employees, not your kids or grandkids.

We wrack our brains for an agency to help with mold and then remember the big deal over anthrax. Who handled the anthrax-contaminated Federal Government buildings? The National Institute for Occupational Health and Safety (NIOSH). But state schools are not Federal Government buildings. NIOSH can't help.

Surprisingly, no U.S. government agency has the responsibility or the ability to regulate indoor pollutants in our schools or homes. And as of now, no U.S. government agency has any significant efforts underway to study indoor pollutants such as neurotoxins from common indoor molds. But there is some hope.

CDC, USDA Recognize the Dangers of Mycotoxins

In March, 2005, the Centers for Disease Control issued warnings about the potential biowarfare threat posed by mycotoxins (mold toxins):

- ☑ *Mycotoxins might be weaponized and dispersed through the air or mixed in food or beverages.*
- ☑ *Dermal exposure leads to burning pain, redness, and blisters, and oral exposure leads to vomiting and diarrhea.*
- ☑ *Dermal exposure leads to burning pain, redness, and blisters, and oral exposure leads to vomiting and diarrhea.*
- ☑ *Ocular exposure might result in blurred vision, and inhalational exposure might cause nasal irritation and cough.*

☑ *Systemic symptoms can develop with all routes of exposure and might include weakness, ataxia, hypotension, coagulopathy, and death.*

The full CDC release is located in the Appendix. In Chapter 3, we discuss mycotoxins in biowarfare in greater detail. We cover research on mold toxins in biowarfare recently published by the U.S. Surgeon General.

The USDA has also conducted a tremendous amount of research on the dangers of food tainted with mycotoxins. The Appendix also includes a 2005 report on mycotoxin contamination in cattle and milk products.

Symptoms from mycotoxin exposure in cattle may include: "reduced production, reduced feed consumption, intermittent diarrhea (sometimes with bloody or dark manure), reduced feed intake, rough hair coat, reduced reproductive performance including irregular estrus cycles, embryonic mortalities, pregnant cows showing estrus, and decreased conception rates."

The report is a serious concern to the numerous cattle and dairy farmers in North America that supply our meat and milk. Both the USDA and the CDC reports should silence any skeptics who dare say that mold only causes runny noses. However, the reports are not directly related to mold in schools. Research in the U.S. on adverse health effects from mold-contaminated schools and Sick Buildings simply pales in comparison to the work being done in Europe and Canada.

Healthy Schools in Europe and Canada

Many European countries know that indoor molds in sick buildings are toxic to the nervous system and brain. So they have very strict guidelines for exposure to indoor mold in Europe and Canada.

European governments take sick buildings *seriously*. For example, their procedures for removing material contaminated by indoor mold are similar to the procedures for removing cancer-producing asbestos.

Canadian researchers consider mold in homes second only to the dangers of parents' secondhand cigarette smoke. In Canada, the provincial governments employ occupational mycologists (health professionals with extensive training in molds) to inspect public and private buildings for mold infestation. Canada also has official mold exposure guidelines.

Buildings are required to be evacuated if elevated levels of toxic fungi are detected in the air. Canada has spent tens of millions of dollars on reducing mold in sick buildings, particularly in schools.

In Germany, government researchers have been studying the effects of toxic molds on animal foods and farmers for more than thirty years. They now have turned their significant research skills to studying Indoor Air Quality and the effect mold toxins have on people who live, work, or go to school in sick buildings.

German scientists have learned that:

☑ A significant number of people exposed to toxins in mold–contaminated buildings will develop acute neurotoxicity (their nervous systems will be poisoned);

☑ Common indoor molds found in water-damaged environments produce toxins that include neurotoxins. Dangerous molds are not limited to the less commonly found *Stachybotrys* (black mold); and

☑ No other common sources of neurotoxins exist in the sick person's environment besides those produced by molds.

German scientists have concluded that molds commonly found in Sick Buildings can and do cause brain trauma and brain disorders.

In other words, respiratory and immuno-suppressive disorders are not the only harmful effects of mold.

EPA Scientist's Cure Covered-Up in the U.S.!

At the EPA, Dr. Kenneth Hudnell is a lead scientist studying biotoxins. Dr. Hudnell was in the news in the 1990s for discovering why so many people were getting very sick when swimming in lakes and streams in Maryland. He found the water was contaminated with neurotoxins produced by algae-like *Pfiesteria*.

Dr. Hudnell and his prolific colleague, Dr. Ritchie Shoemaker, cured people suffering from acute neurotoxicity and dozens of other symptoms resulting from contact with *Pfiesteria* biotoxins. Hudnell and Shoemaker proved that patients' neurological symptoms can be reversed with the toxin-binding medicine called Cholestyramine (CSM).

Cholestyramine binds mold toxins in the bowels, which allows them to be permanently excreted from the body.

CSM was already an established FDA-approved treatment for reducing high levels of cholesterol. CSM was known to bind cholesterol in the bowels so it could be excreted in the stool.

Neurotoxins from mold and *Pfiesteria*, it turns out, have binding properties similar to cholesterol. Cholestyramine will also bind to *Pfiesteria*-produced toxins in a person's digestive system and, as with cholesterol, such toxins will be excreted and permanently removed.

Dr. Hudnell reported that some people who got sick from exposure to *Pfiesteria* quickly recovered without treatment. Many did not get sick at all. However, a significant percent of sick people could not recover without receiving the Cholestyramine toxin-binding treatment. Most of the people recovered quickly once the toxin-binding treatment started.

People with mold biotoxin-related illness from homes or schools, according to Dr. Hudnell, also had success with Cholestyramine.

The latest scientific evidence from these researchers now tells us why some people exposed to toxic indoor mold or *Pfiesteria* get sick and some do not. Some people (approximately 1 in 4) have a genetic predisposition to such toxicity; that is, their genes make them more susceptible to the poisons.

The people who don't get sick are able to quickly remove these biotoxins from their systems. Toxins are removed from the blood by the liver, kidney or antibodies. So as long as someone is not exposed to *high* mold toxin levels, their bodies can function properly. However, people who are susceptible to the toxins cannot remove even *moderate* amounts of toxins efficiently.

You might ask yourself why we don't we hear more about this EPA toxin-binding cure. The reason is simple: to promote the cure, you need to accept that indoor mold causes more than a runny nose and red eyes. There is wide-spread reluctance by many businesses, school boards, drug companies, insurance companies, and government entities to accept that such mold toxins exist and can make people sick.

Arm Yourself With Research

While there have been hundreds of medical and scientific studies linking mold toxins to ill human health, two recent studies, one funded by the EPA and one funded by the National Academy of Science, are really starting to turn heads. The EPA publication is the first government-funded research that warns clinicians to be on the lookout for kids that may be suffering from neurological illnesses due to mold toxins. The entire work may be downloaded for free from the EPA web site:

http://oehc.uchc.edu/clinser/MOLD%20GUIDE.pdf

The National Academy of Science book, *Damp Indoor Spaces*[6], details numerous studies showing that molds common in water-damaged homes can produce biotoxins, including neurotoxins. The animal studies report that the toxins can even cause death.

Mold Professional Recommendations

While most Americans may not have heard about this toxin-binding cure, if you are in the mold remediation business, you most likely are aware of toxin-binding therapy.

Mold testers and remediators get exposed to mold biotoxins regularly and many "swear by" toxin-binders to keep them healthy.

Prescription Treatment

Mold professionals often take Cholestyramine (CSM) before and after mold jobs. And since toxic mold exposure can be accompanied by fungal growth in the sinuses, as well as fungal infections in the throat, an antifungal agent such as Difulcan is occasionally taken by mold remediators only if sinus or throat symptoms persist in a mold-free environment.

Many other treatment options are used for people who have had long-term exposure to mold that causes a domino effect in the body including: increased inflammation, autoimmunity, hormonal abnormalities, and blood thickening.

Another possible prescription treatment is the use of Actos, which is a diabetes medication. The *New England Journal of Medicine* shows Actos has the ability to turn off inflammation chemicals. Dr. Ritchie Shoemaker, the author of *Mold Warriors*, has been successfully using this treatment for many years.

Non-Prescription Treatment

Whether or not the following treatments are as effective as prescription treatments is unknown. But some mold remediation contractors use these non-prescription treatments both for prevention and for treatment. Use these at your own risk. None of these are FDA-approved and it is considered legally improper to make an exact health claim. Dr. Rosen is merely sharing his experience in conjunction with information from veteran mold inspectors and remediators.

A few studies seem to show Chitosan has potential as a mold toxin binder. Chitosan is commonly known as a “fat binder” and is found in many weight-loss formulas. While some mold remediators use Chitosan, Dr. Shoemaker has not found it effective and only recommends Cholestyramine (or rarely, a weaker medication, Welchol). Activated pharmaceutical-grade charcoal capsules also may have some use as a toxin binder. Studies show that charcoal binds some mold toxins but is poor at binding others. Both Chitosan and activated charcoal are available at most health food stores.

The inflammation that always accompanies chronic mold toxin exposure is occasionally treated with over-the-counter products such as Advil and Nuprin. Yet be aware these may have side effects on the stomach, intestines and kidneys. If you need them routinely, remove all mold exposures and seek out a mold knowledgeable physician, since it is unwise to use a Band-Aid to hide ongoing mold toxin inflammation damage.

Some studies also report Omega-3 fatty acid fish oil supplements and I.V. magnesium are useful in reducing inflammation when taken at high doses.

Since Dr. Schaller has over fifty treatment innovations, throughout this book we will discuss a wide range of treatment options utilizing both traditional and progressive medicine. These include new medications, old medications with new uses, herbal options, special delivery options for anti-inflammatory nutrients, and many other healing tools.

Fixing Mold in your Home

The first medical treatment for mold illness is finding and removing the mold. Period.

The EPA guide to mold in your home is clearly written and a good reference. See "A Brief Guide to Mold, Moisture, and Your Home" at *www.epa.gov/mold.*

It is important to understand that visible mold is more of a problem to people's health than mold *fully sealed* inside of walls. Regardless of the mold's location, the first thing to do when people are sick is to eliminate the water source so that mold growth stops. After that, eliminate all visible and easily accessible mold. Mold spores and mold toxin-containing dust become air-borne when disturbed, so you want to be careful not to disturb mold. Never brush or sweep mold or direct a fan or AC duct toward mold growth.

After removing all visible mold, there may still be some mold inside the wall or ceiling.

- ☑ Make sure that all openings to the ceiling and wall cavities are sealed.
- ☑ Make sure you put a MERV 11 air filter in your AC.
- ☑ Make sure to turn the AC FAN ON (not AUTO) to continuously filter the air.

If you follow this procedure and have eliminated the water source—even though you don't eliminate all hidden mold—the airborne mold (mold in the air your breath that makes you sick) will usually be reduced to such an extent that most people will no longer get sick.

CHAPTER 3

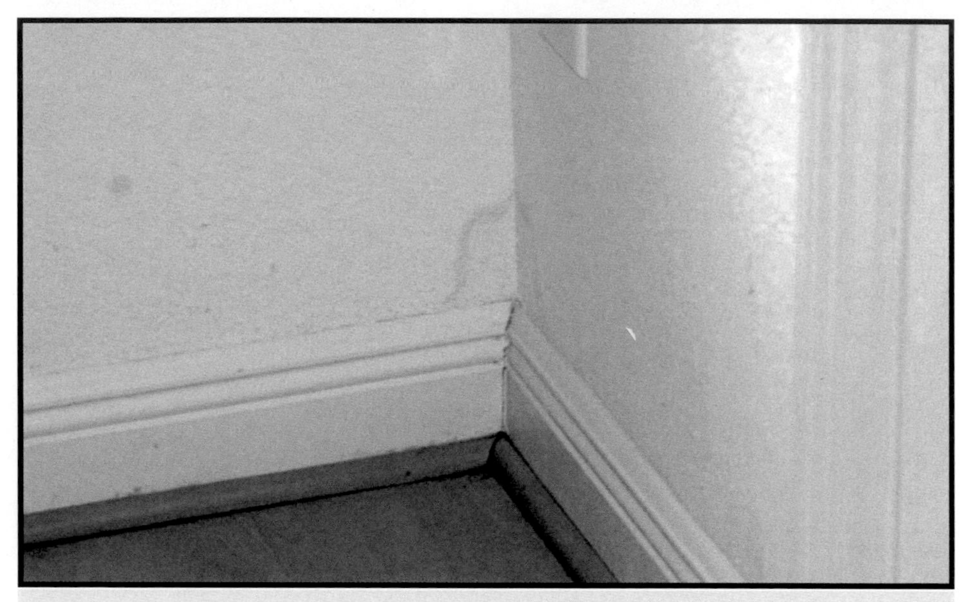

See the next page to find out what was hidden behind this wall with a small water stain.

Sick Buildings and Sick People: What We Can Learn from U.S. Army Biowarfare Research[7,8]

While the focus of U.S. Army research on mold toxins is in regard to Biowarfare, much of the findings are directly applicable to Sick Building Syndrome. Army Biowarfare research helps us answer the following questions:

- ☑ How can mold toxin exposures make someone sick beyond allergic and asthma problems?
- ☑ How people can be treated for such exposures?

Introduction to Mold Neurotoxins

People are still surprised to learn that many mold biotoxins are actually neurotoxic. In other words, chemicals produced by indoor molds can directly harm brain cells. Perhaps the most well-known neurotoxins are released by marine bacteria. During the warm summer months, algae-like organisms "bloom" or reproduce in large numbers, creating a "red tide." The huge quantities of neurotoxins released by these organisms make the waters unsafe for humans and kill tons of fish as well as mammals like manatees and dolphins.

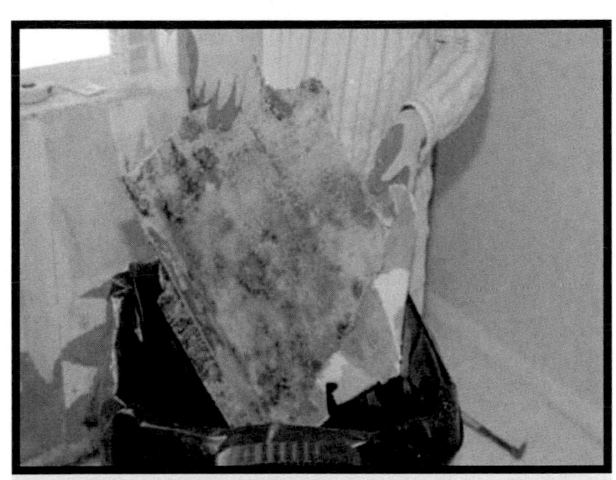

Hidden mold may be extensive even though only a slight glimpse is indicated on the outer wall. This was caused by a leaking sink. Indoor levels of toxic mold were **100,000** times higher than the outdoor levels.

See the EPA web site at *http://www.epa.gov/cyano_habs_symposium/* for additional information on neurotoxin-producing bacteria.

Mushrooms, a close relative to mold, produce the well-known neurotoxin, LSD or "acid."

It should not be surprising then that mold, again a close relative to mushrooms, also can produce certain toxins. And though these mold toxins may be directed at molds' competitors (bacteria and other molds), many are very potent and can affect people.

The mold toxin trichothecene is often found in water-damaged homes, schools and offices (Sick Buildings). Trichothecene is a known neurotoxin and produced by *Stachybotrys* (The "Black Mold"), *Fusaria*, and *Trichoderma*—some sixty molds in total.

The Use of Mold Toxins in War

The Army reports that trichothecene was a biological warfare agent in the "yellow rain" attacks in Southeast Asia. This resulted in a great deal of Army-funded research on trichothecene and its effects on humans. The research is now declassified and available from the Surgeon General's office.[3]

This Army research is very important because it documents that mycotoxin exposures:

☑ Were tested on laboratory animals and, surprisingly, humans as well; and

☑ Cause not only respiratory damage from inhalation, but also neurological damage to humans.

Human Guinea Pigs

Army research reports that in the late 1970s and early 1980s, a form of trichothecene was tested on humans! Due to the debilitating effects of trichothecene on rapidly proliferating cells, researchers thought the toxins might stall tumor growth. As a result, a test group of cancer patients were given intravenous doses of trichothecene. According to researchers, the patients experienced the common symptoms of neurotoxin poisoning: nausea, burning erythema (red skin), confusion, coordination trouble, and low blood pressure. Testing of trichothecene as an anticancer drug was abandoned due the life-threatening symptoms and insignificant anti-tumor activity.

<u>The Army's research helps dispel some common myths.</u>

Myth #1: Mold poisoning is a "fad" or scare tactic used by the mold industry to generate business.

Myth #2: Mycotoxins affect only the respiratory system and there is no evidence that mycotoxins affect other parts of the body, such as the human brain.

Myth #3: There is no cure.

Exposure through Eating, Breathing or Touching Mold Toxins

Mycotoxins can enter your body through the skin, mouth or lungs. Army researchers were very interested in studying how the routes of exposure determine toxicity levels. Routes of exposure in Sick Buildings are similar to exposure routes from Biowarfare attacks and can include:

- Swallowing via nasal mucous or saliva as a result of being in mold-contaminated air;
- Absorption through the skin (e.g., sitting in a chair covered with mycotoxins); or
- Breathing toxin-contaminated air.

Army Biowarfare research found that any of these routes of mycotoxin exposure can cause severe effects such as vomiting, nausea, diarrhea, dizziness, and central nervous system toxicity, which can lead to memory loss, lassitude, sexual dysfunction, vision impairment, and low blood pressure.

However, some symptoms are route-dependent. For instance, skin exposure can lead to painful inflammation, rashes and even skin death.

Route-specific symptoms also can occur from inhalation. In fact, aerosolized trichothecenes can lead to severe respiratory disease and even death.

Cleaning the Body of Mold Toxins

The healthy human body will begin detoxifying itself soon after mycotoxin exposure, unless the exposure is high enough to cause immediate death. Mycotoxins are rapidly metabolized by the kidney and liver and then excreted in urine and feces.

Army recommended treatments are as follows:

- Wash contaminated skin within 4 to 6 hours of exposure. This can remove up to 98% of the toxins residing on the skin;
- Take activated charcoal pills, which are stocked in military hospitals worldwide. Activated charcoal binds to the toxins in bile and helps flush them out of the body.

Currently, a significant amount of work is being done in Europe on toxin-binding therapy for curing farm animals poisoned by mold toxins in their feeds.[9,10,11,12,13]

Toxin binders such as Cholestyramine are now being prescribed by physicians (not just veterinarians) involved in treating mold-related illnesses. Plus, some mold remediators routinely take a wide range of toxin binders to prevent health problems from mold toxin exposure.

Conclusions

In conclusion, Army Biowarfare research can shed light on several important topics related to mold toxin contamination:

- ☑ Mold toxin exposure can produce neurotoxic affects in people.
- ☑ Toxin binders can help people exposed to mold toxins return to health.

Dr. Schaller is working on a book that compares dozens of mold binders, mold toxin denaturing options, and ways to enhance the body's own toxin-removal mechanisms.

> The complete Chapter 34 of the U.S. Army Research on Mycotoxins can be found in the Surgeon General's report on Mycotoxins at:
>
> *http://www.nbe-ced.org/SiteContent/HomePage/WhatsNew/MedAspects/Ch-34electrv699.pdf*

CHAPTER 4

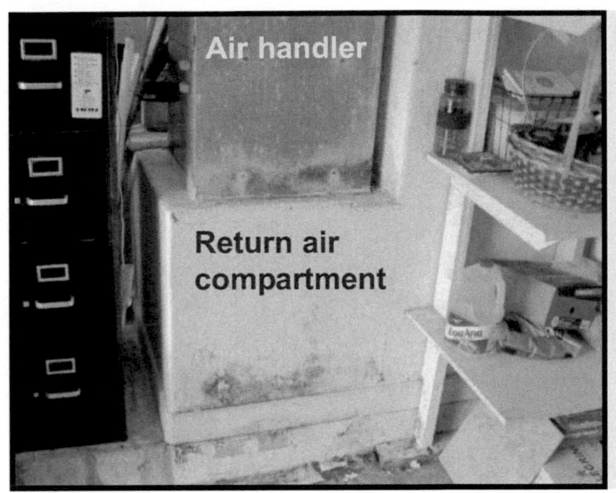

This photo shows a problem air-handler in a garage. A cabinet up against the AC unit base (return air plenum) hid the mold and water stains from sight. Everyone in the house was sick. The inside of the AC return air compartment was black with toxic mold. This was easily replaced with new by the AC service. Within weeks, everyone returned to health without the need for toxin-binding therapy.

Mold's Effect on Emotions

The emotions coming from the brain are very closely tied to the functioning of the body. Any abnormality in the long-term health of the body will have an effect on the brain, particularly on the emotional state of a child or parent. A very common manifestation of mold toxin exposure is emotional struggles.

Day in and day out you may be seeing the effects of indoor mold on people you know without even realizing it. You might think that your spouse, significant other, child, relatives, siblings, friends, boss, co-workers, or neighbors do not "seem right" to you.

Since indoor mold growth is so common, mold toxin exposure should be considered as a possible cause of any unexplained emotional or personality change.

Traditional physicians have little time to discuss subtle personality changes, but they now have access to many analytical tools to help diagnose the impact of mold toxins on the body. These tests measure mold toxin exposure and have nothing to do with allergic reactions to mold. Since allergic reactions to mold are reasonably well understood by traditional medicine, they are not covered in this book.

A small sample of important lab tests available for any physician to order would include: MSH, VIP, VEGF, C3a, and leptin (all discussed in detail in Ch. 16); the visual contrast sensitivity test (Ch. 11); DNA profiling of nasal fluids (showing the DNA of molds breathed in, as studied in recent EPA research and discussed earlier on page ii); and many others discussed throughout this book.

Many readily measurable indicators become abnormal with mold exposure. These indicators return to normal following treatment and mold remediation (Ch. 15) and/or the use of special MERV 11 air filters (Ch. 14), which continuously reduce the level of mold spores in a contaminated environment.

For example, MSH is one hormone that is commonly abnormal in people ill from mold toxin exposure. Abnormal MSH levels can cause personality changes such as irritability, restlessness, boredom, and slow cognition. This should be no surprise since MSH is involved in many functions, including keeping nerves healthy, controlling inflammation, producing natural mood enhancers, and reducing pain.

A physician examining a patient for possible mold illness should not only measure levels of important blood indicators, but also ask if there have been any changes in the patient's emotional state.

Boredom

John was not enjoying his recent move. He did not like his new home or his new school. When he admitted to feeling intensely bored and hopeless, his mother, whose aunt had committed suicide, jumped into action. She signed him up for two kinds of traditional therapy, but this did not help much. She next requested a medication trial, and he was very sensitive to 1/8th of the smallest recommended dose. Such extreme sensitivity is a flag for something besides basic major depression. It is a sign that the patient may have excess inflammation, infections such as Lyme or Bartonella (which are rarely detected by lab testing), poor detoxification by the liver, and/or mold biotoxin exposure.

Processing Trauma

Emily's boyfriend cheated on her about nine months ago. She talks about it like it was yesterday. They had only been dating for two months. Her MSH hormone was zero. MSH helps with coping, handling stress, and decreasing pain. Mold toxins are often the cause of this problem as they turn off MSH.

LabCorp of America has a special kit for measuring MSH. It is common to find the critical hormone MSH, with over twenty key body functions, at very low levels when mold contaminates the patient's home or school. Probably millions of Americans have abnormally low MSH due to mold biotoxin poisoning.

The fact that many doctors do not test for this critical hormone is amazing. Instead, they unsuccessfully treat mold symptoms–but not the cause–with new or different drugs or order a string of different allergy tests.

Excess Irritability

Evan is a GYM teacher at a local public school. He has slowly become more hostile over the last six years. He scares his wife with his temper. She reports at times he "shorts out." He is unsettled when trying to deal with more than one topic or activity at a time. Occasionally, modest sounds, bright lights, or people talking loudly make him very angry. If his children speak simultaneously, it seems to cut him with an invisible knife. Sometimes he yells at them so loudly that he can be heard outside the house fifty feet away.

Evan is very hostile at the end of a workweek and seems "thin skinned" with little emotional reserve for the weekend. He improved fifty percent with an antidepressant, but further dose increases did not result in further improvements. A few parents have complained about his belittling comments toward their children.

He was better during the summer when school was not in session. When he returned to school in late August, his mood worsened. His wife's diary noted the change. Was the problem related to job stress? But this made little sense since Evan really loved his job.

His wife went to Evan's job one weekend and took seven swab samples from moisture-damaged walls and cabinets in her husband's work area. He was literally working in a leaky greenhouse full of mold! Further, since the school could not afford to run and maintain the AC units, it had weeks and months at well over 65% indoor humidity, which is the threshold over which molds will thrive. Evan is currently in litigation with the school district to have the school building fixed.

Regressed Feelings & Thoughts

Mary feels a new, strong need to be closer to her family, especially her mother, for unknown reasons. She is "clingy" with her family and needs more affection and time alone with her mother. Nothing in her life circumstances can adequately explain this change. The cause is routinely missed by sincere therapists. Mary's roof leak led to moisture and mold under her floral wallpaper. The inflammation from the mold toxins caused regression and immaturity.

Kevin used to be moderately open-minded, but now he seems to think in the black or white manner of a child. This is a type of regressed thinking resulting from mold toxin exposure. Specifically, people are smart or stupid, good or bad, mature or childish, generous or stingy. People are either for him or against him, supportive or drags. But as we know, people usually do not fit these black or white labels. Kevin's basement has regularly leaked, and he is casual about the mold in his basement. His thinking is simplistic: "Mold is just mold," he says. But his lab results point to mold toxin exposure as the most likely reason for his emotional distress as well as his recent weight gain.

New Anxiety

Adam has attended the same parochial school for five years. He knows the location of every class, as well as the names of all the teachers and staff. It has felt like a second home for years. Recently, it has started to feel uncomfortable to him. Although he is in the sixth grade, and is used to feeling like a "big kid" at school, he has a new shyness.

He did not go out for the school play or track because he did not want to be "watched." This was new.

His home has moderate mold, and his blood tests showed he is part of the twenty-five percent of Americans with genes that prevent his body from effectively removing mold biotoxins.

Agitation and Panic

"When I stand before my class," Mr. Jenkins said, "I feel like I could jump out of my skin." Mr. Jenkins had been teaching high school successfully for almost twenty years, so this was unusual.

"I must be burned out," he said. "I likely need a vacation."

He had been transferred to another school, and he reported having panic attacks when he was asked to talk with parents at parent-teacher meetings.

"The parents expect perfect teaching in this district. I fear I just will not be able to cut it."

Mr. Jenkins had been well received every year by faculty, administration, students, and parents. He was an exceptional teacher.

One of the school employees recently finished a short class on mold in schools. He took a few samples for Mr. Jenkins. He cut a piece from an air filter, took a dust sample from the AC duct, and took three air samples from suspicious locations. Instead of finding a mix of typical outdoor molds, sample results showed high numbers of several biotoxin-producing molds. Seven other teachers also reported symptoms common to mold toxin exposure, and eventually the school had some modest remediation and special mold spore cleaning done.

After the remediation, Mr. Jenkins had about a sixty percent decrease in his panic and agitation, but transferred to a new charter school the following year. He had no hope the school would fully repair the mold problem and tried charcoal capsules that he was able to buy without a prescription. They did not have much effect.

He read about how Cholestyramine capsules bind to mold toxins and, during the summer, started on an aggressive dose of Cholestyramine under a doctor's supervision. He has not had any symptoms at the new school.

CHAPTER 5

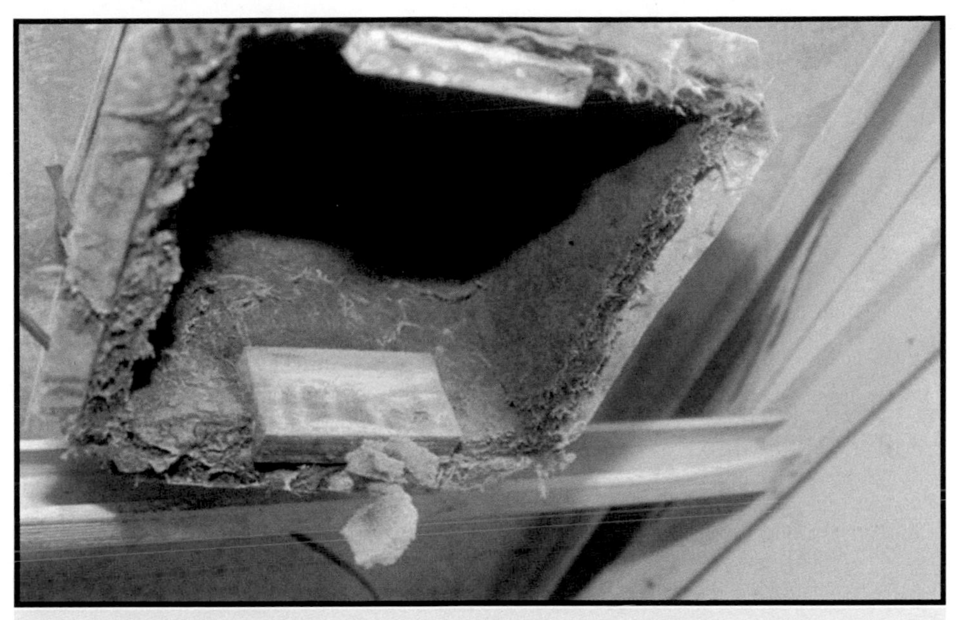

This grossly contaminated air duct is proof of why quality air filters should be used to keep ducts clean of dust. The dust grows mold. No Dust = No Mold. In this case, the ducts were so bad that the ceiling of the home had to be removed and all the ducts replaced. That sure is expensive compared to changing your air filters every month or two!

Mold Spores: Armed and Dangerous

Molds are fungi that feed off of a host. For mold, that host might be a moist section of your carpet, a wall in your bathroom, or the school library. Molds have defense mechanisms to protect their seeds (spores) from competitors and enemies. Competitors and enemies include other molds and bacteria, all battling over the same patch of moist carpet, humid air conditioning duct, or damp wallboard in your home or your child's school.

Some molds use a form of chemical warfare to protect their seeds just as poisonous bacteria such as botulism and anthrax do. These chemical protectors are called *bio*toxins because they are toxins produced by living organisms (*bio* = living). These biotoxins, unfortunately, can be breathed, swallowed and absorbed through your skin. Over extended periods of time, children and even adults exposed to these toxins can also be affected by them.

"Don't eat that!" we warn, as a child leans down to pick a mushroom or fungus. Every child learns that many mushrooms are poisonous when eaten. Is the fungi biotoxin defense working? You bet!

While you can teach your kids not to eat poisonous mushrooms, toxic mold spores are harder to avoid. They are invisible. When inhaled, these spores, or their dust-bound biotoxins, land inside the sinuses or on wet lung tissue and must be quickly removed by the body's defense mechanisms. Fungi don't grow in the lungs or sinuses of healthy individuals because our immune system removes them. But when you or your child inhales toxin-covered mold spores, the toxins on the spore are left behind even if the spore is cleared from the body. This is particularly problematic in young children because children do not have fully developed immune systems.

The best-known example of a biotoxin from a mold is Penicillin. An "antibiotic" is a substance toxic to bacteria.[14]

Penicillium is one of the molds that typically will colonize humid or moist buildings. *Aspergillus* and *Stachybotrys* are two other molds that are often found in sick buildings. While *Stachybotrys* is only found when there is/was ample water damage, *Aspergillus* and *Penicillium* do not need much water to grow. In fact, they actually can grow and produce toxins with only high humidity.

These three problem molds found in sick buildings all produce toxins that are poisonous when ingested or casually inhaled as your child sits at school or plays in your basement.

The discovery of the antibiotic penicillin (an antibacterial toxin) from toxic mold has proven a godsend for humankind. However, toxic mold as a result of indoor humidity problems or water damage in today's "tight" homes, schools or offices is growing into a plague. And since one of its symptoms is decreased insight and decreased body awareness, it is a stealth plague.

Just How Dangerous Are Molds?

Some mold toxins from *Penicillium*, *Aspergillus* and *Stachybotrys* are very dangerous. Their toxins harm human respiratory systems and immune systems, but can also affect any organ in the body, including the human brain.

The effects of mold toxins on children include memory loss, learning disabilities, attention deficit disorders (ADD or ADHD), headaches, moodiness, oppositionality, anxiety, boredom, insomnia, addictive behavior, impulsivity, excess dependence, fatigue, vision problems, narcissism, reactivity, sexual dysfunction, and some loss of coordination.

Unfortunately, pediatricians, family doctors, teachers, psychologists, and child psychiatrists are not trained to realize that mold toxins can easily cause these problems. So their solutions, which are geared toward treating the symptoms, are only partly effective.

Furthermore, with prolonged exposure to mold neurotoxins, these problems can turn into permanent disabilities and scar the brain. Neurotoxins from toxic molds are facts accepted by the Food and Drug Administration, the Environmental Protection Agency, and other U.S. government agencies. What is new is just how common these toxic molds are in damp buildings and the direct link between mold neurotoxins and hundreds of child problems.

Are we saying that neurotoxins from mold in sick schools could cause or exacerbate your child's reading disability or ADD? Absolutely!

One in four children is sensitive to indoor mold toxins. Mold toxins can worsen a child's medical or psychiatric illnesses. A child with asthma, allergies, ADHD, or even shyness will suffer more if exposed to indoor mold. Sometimes, mold is the only cause of these problems.

Do you still doubt that mold cannot be toxic? Mold toxins have been weaponized in Iraq and Russia in the past. These are "war mold" toxins, not molds for making beer and cheese.

"War molds" are commonly found in sick buildings and homes all around you and around the world. They are making people ill in mysterious ways that are routinely not properly diagnosed.

An Idiot's Guide to Mold

While the many "Idiot's Guides" books are meant to educate, we want to discuss the actual comments about indoor mold spoken by verifiable idiots.

Some argue against mold as the culprit for sick schools, sick students, sick offices, and sick employees. Some write it off as "media hype."

Media Hype

"We've always had mold in the world. The real problem is that the media blows everything out of proportion." Yes, some indoor mold has always been with us, but not in the concentrations breathed today. The increase in mold-related health problems is directly due to our breathing more mold-contaminated indoor air.

- ☑ The U.S. government reports that asthma in children is 300% more common than it was twenty-five years ago. Doctors have been able to diagnose a person suffocating from asthma for the past quarter century. It is hardly an invisible illness. Does media hype explain this massive increase in asthma that is due to poor indoor air quality?
- ☑ Our children spend more and more time indoors, up to 90% of their lives. And tighter, less leaky, more "energy efficient" schools, homes and offices mean less clean fresh air that would flush out toxin-filled air. Recycling stale indoor air is less costly than bringing in outside air that must be warmed, cooled, and/or dehumidified. As a result, there are more sick schools and more kids sick from attending them.
- ☑ When plaster walls were replaced with drywall, mold found a new food source. While plaster is inorganic and mold cannot grow on it, drywall is made with cellulose (paper) and is a very good food source for mold when wet.

Mold Toxins in Blood or Urine

Directly finding mold biotoxins in human blood or urine is inherently difficult because the mold toxins are so powerful that only minute levels in the human body make us sick. Physicians currently do not have routine lab tests to measure the diverse types of mold toxins people acquire in a moldy building. While scientists can measure toxins on the mold spores or in the mold bodies themselves, low toxin levels in human blood cannot be readily measured. Therefore, some physicians claim that they do not actually exist.

Sick schools, homes and offices are typically infected with dozens of species of molds, and at least three or four of these produce toxins. And a single toxin-producing mold species will produce quite an assortment of different toxins.

Due to the multitude of toxins, determining the specific mold toxins causing a specific symptom is not an easy task. As a general rule, we believe that most mold-related sickness is likely due to a combination of toxins.

One famous toxic mold is the toxic "black mold," *Stachybotrys*. It produces extensive toxins, many of which are not yet understood. Compounding the identification process, toxin-producing molds also produce other chemicals that are active in the human body. These chemicals function as immunosuppressive agents, which leave a person more susceptible to illness, but are not actually classified as "toxins."

Threshold Limits

One of the unknowns in mold toxin medical care is the threshold amount required to make someone sick. Determining what levels of mold are dangerous is difficult. Since, of course, studies on humans are unethical, most of the research is based on rat studies. You cannot poison people to advance medicine.

Since you cannot ask a rat about a headache, scientists study the effects of mold toxins on rats by determining at what point the rats die or their brain starts to bleed. This is what non-clinical scientists can easily measure. Of course, a much higher dose is needed to kill the rat than to make it ill, such as with a headache.

But here is the kicker: because the levels of mold toxins that produce a response (death or brain hemorrhage) in laboratory animal experiments are higher than the levels typically found in homes or schools, some people think mold toxins can't hurt you.

This reasoning is dangerous and laughable but strongly supported by certain people and organizations that care more about money and status quo than your child's health.

They are masters at twisting and turning information to suit their needs and do not care who suffers as a result. Similarly, for many years arguments were made that defended cigarette smoking. But eventually the tide turned and we now accept the widespread research showing that cigarette smoke can kill. The tide is starting to turn on recognizing the dangers of indoor mold.

And the longer this debate continues, the longer our children's health will suffer, as will their education. To a great degree, it is not old books or substandard teachers that are causing America's youth to underperform in the classroom. Rather, it is old leaky school buildings contaminated with mold that are reducing the functioning of both students and teachers, making learning harder. Indoor mold toxicity is the asbestos of the new millennium. And it is in 30% of U.S. structures.

CHAPTER 6

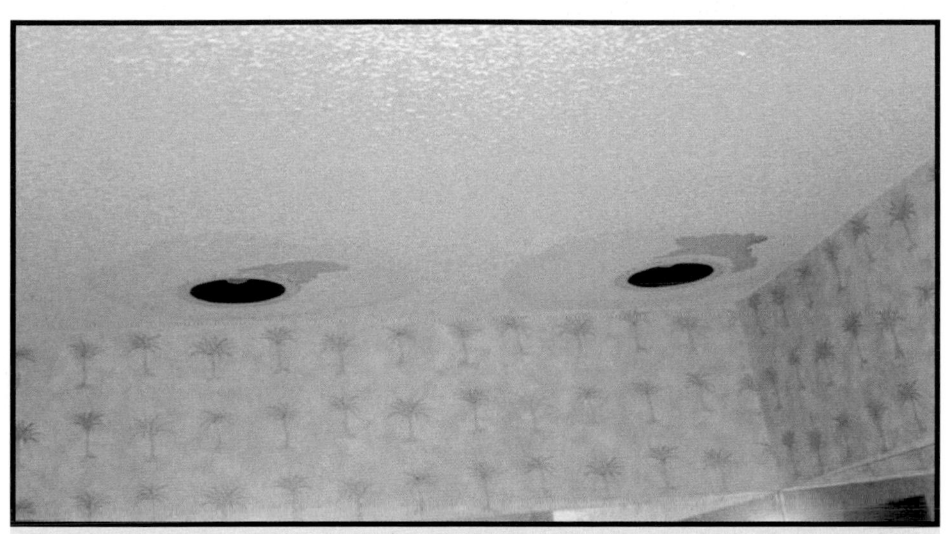

Serious roof leaks caused massive mold problems in the attic that could not be cleaned up due to inaccessible attic space. These old fashioned recessed lights were not air tight. When the homeowners replaced them with modern air-tight fixtures, the odors and mold inside the house from the attic dissipated and the occupants returned to health.

How Common Mold Toxins Hurt Your Child & You

A List of Symptoms, Signs and Body Parts Hurt by Mold

Parents may wonder if their child's emotional or health troubles come from mold toxins. We have reviewed over two hundred articles on mold symptoms, and below we list the most common effects of mold on the mind and body. No one suffers from all of these symptoms and some are only present in very severe exposures.

Even modest mold exposure can significantly affect relationships, as well as school or work performance. Mold chemicals can enter the air from hidden mold sources with the mere vibration of a stereo or opening and closing a door. The toxic mold chemicals are then dispersed all over a school or home. Once they enter your lungs or are swallowed via your nasal fluids or saliva, they will travel all over the body.

If sensitive people are exposed to toxic mold, they can experience some combination of *hundreds* of different body problems.

Please remember that if you spend any time in a musty location or a place with visible indoor mold, you will be exposed to mold toxins. High levels of exposure overwhelm everyone. Modest mold toxin exposure will bother the 25% of the population that is sensitive. These sensitive individuals need to be extra careful with mold because they do not remove the toxins from their systems as quickly as non-sensitive people. The toxins then tend to build up in their bodies. Sensitive people must be sure to live in a home that has no hidden indoor mold. Furthermore, they cannot go to school or work in moldy buildings.

Unlike with typical viral or bacterial infections, there is no single test that will show if your child is ill from mold biotoxin exposure. But one "test" is simply comparing your child to healthy peers. Look over the list at the end of this chapter and see how many symptoms fit you or your child. Mark each one that fits. The number does not have to be extreme to indicate mold toxin exposure. Take note of any symptoms present in your child for at least one month, paying special attention to symptoms that are more noticeable in your child than in healthy peers. But do not compare your child to other children going to the same moldy school or living in the same moldy home! They may all be sick from mold.

Quick Confirmation

The confirmation of the diagnosis can sometimes come from a fast cure. Sometimes removal from the offending location, such as during a long vacation, or the use of mold toxin-binding medication such as Cholestyramine, shows that mold was the likely cause.

Many toxic mold patients can have ten or more of these symptoms. Exposed children can report a lower number because they are poor at reporting subtle body and mind changes. Keep in mind the principle of "insight impairment" that should be assumed in mold illness. In other words, mold illness may blind the affected child or adult to their symptoms until they have massive undeniable deficits.

The Vacation Test

Sometimes a child is better on the weekends, during long vacations, or during the summer. Often, this does not mean they hate math, but rather, that they are temporarily removed from a sick school. The return of behavioral, emotional, or learning symptoms after a week back in a moldy school or home is strong evidence of mold toxins.

On the following two pages, you can see how mold toxins adversely affect the various parts of the human body.

THE EFFECT OF INDOOR MOLD ON THE BRAIN

Seizures
Strokes
Obsessive
Trembling
Headaches
Drug abuse
Immaturity
Forgetfulness
Poor memory
Panic Attacks
Disorientation
Trouble learning
Dead creativity
Depression • Anxiety
Poor organization
Eccentric personality
Poor stress coping
Trouble speaking fast
Abnormal reflexes
Mood swings • Mania
Serotonin changes
Trouble finding words
EEG abnormalities
Trouble concentrating
Vocal or Motor Tics
Irritability • Impulsivity
Decreased attention
Decreased productivity
Increased risk taking
Poor insight into illness
Increased narcissism
Increased verbal fighting
Lateness • Poor empathy
Unable to process trauma
Poor boundary awareness
Spacey • Rigidity • Poor insight
Decreased speech smoothness
Edema or swelling in the brain
Scarring of Brain seen on MRI's
Increased alcohol consumption
Trouble with quick mental tasks
Abnormal PET and SPECT scans
Child developmental milestone delays
Highly sensitive to interpersonal problems

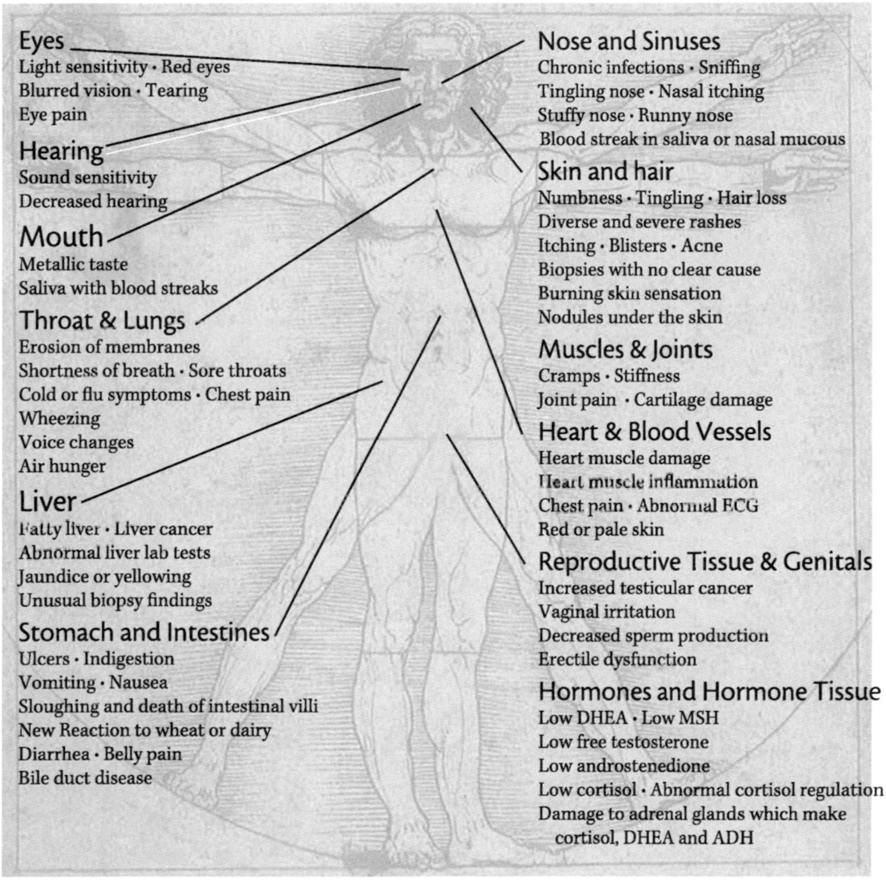

Eyes
Light sensitivity • Red eyes
Blurred vision • Tearing
Eye pain

Hearing
Sound sensitivity
Decreased hearing

Mouth
Metallic taste
Saliva with blood streaks

Throat & Lungs
Erosion of membranes
Shortness of breath • Sore throats
Cold or flu symptoms • Chest pain
Wheezing
Voice changes
Air hunger

Liver
Fatty liver • Liver cancer
Abnormal liver lab tests
Jaundice or yellowing
Unusual biopsy findings

Stomach and Intestines
Ulcers • Indigestion
Vomiting • Nausea
Sloughing and death of intestinal villi
New Reaction to wheat or dairy
Diarrhea • Belly pain
Bile duct disease

Nose and Sinuses
Chronic infections • Sniffing
Tingling nose • Nasal itching
Stuffy nose • Runny nose
Blood streak in saliva or nasal mucous

Skin and hair
Numbness • Tingling • Hair loss
Diverse and severe rashes
Itching • Blisters • Acne
Biopsies with no clear cause
Burning skin sensation
Nodules under the skin

Muscles & Joints
Cramps • Stiffness
Joint pain • Cartilage damage

Heart & Blood Vessels
Heart muscle damage
Heart muscle inflammation
Chest pain • Abnormal ECG
Red or pale skin

Reproductive Tissue & Genitals
Increased testicular cancer
Vaginal irritation
Decreased sperm production
Erectile dysfunction

Hormones and Hormone Tissue
Low DHEA • Low MSH
Low free testosterone
Low androstenedione
Low cortisol • Abnormal cortisol regulation
Damage to adrenal glands which make cortisol, DHEA and ADH

CHAPTER 7

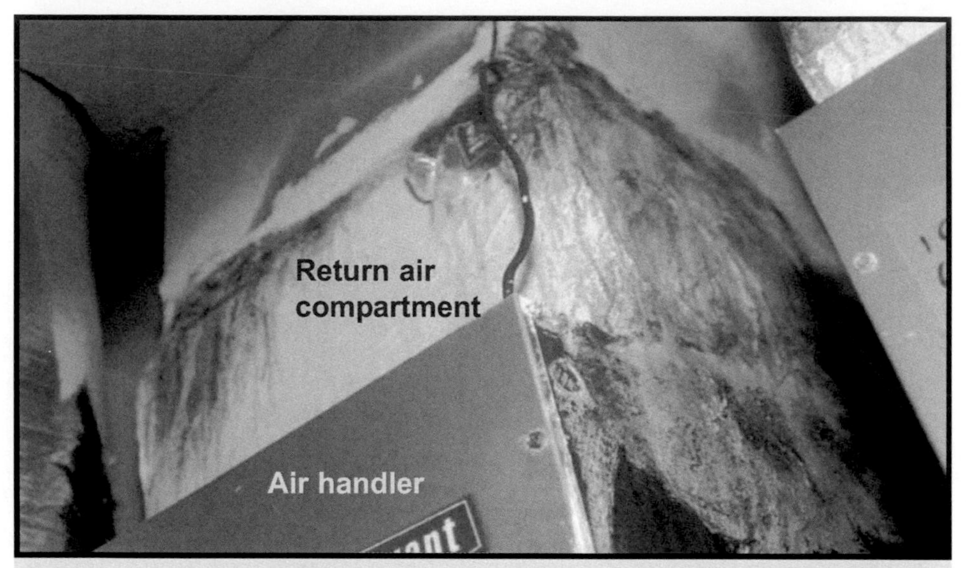

Moist air from the attic leaks into the house and condenses on the cool air handler surface causing mold. This is a very common construction defect. The wife is very sick, while the husband is unaffected. They are suing the builder. The builder claims that this is a maintenance problem, which of course it is not. The house is only 3 years old.

A Brief History of Mold's Effects on Children and Families

Sick Houses in Biblical Times

Sick Buildings actually were recognized by the Law of Moses thousands of years ago. The Bible clearly describes mold infestation of a house. The following passage gives a description of the problem, how to detect and confirm it by inspection, and how to fix it:

The LORD said to Moses and Aaron, "When you enter the land of Canaan, which I am giving you as your possession ... and a spreading mildew [is] in a house in that land, the owner of the house must go and tell the priest, "I have seen something that looks like mildew in my house..." The priest is to go and inspect the house. He is to examine the mildew on the walls ... the priest shall return and inspect the house.

If the mildew has spread on the walls, he is to order that the contaminated stones be torn out and thrown into an unclean place outside of town... (Excerpts from Leviticus 14.33-48)

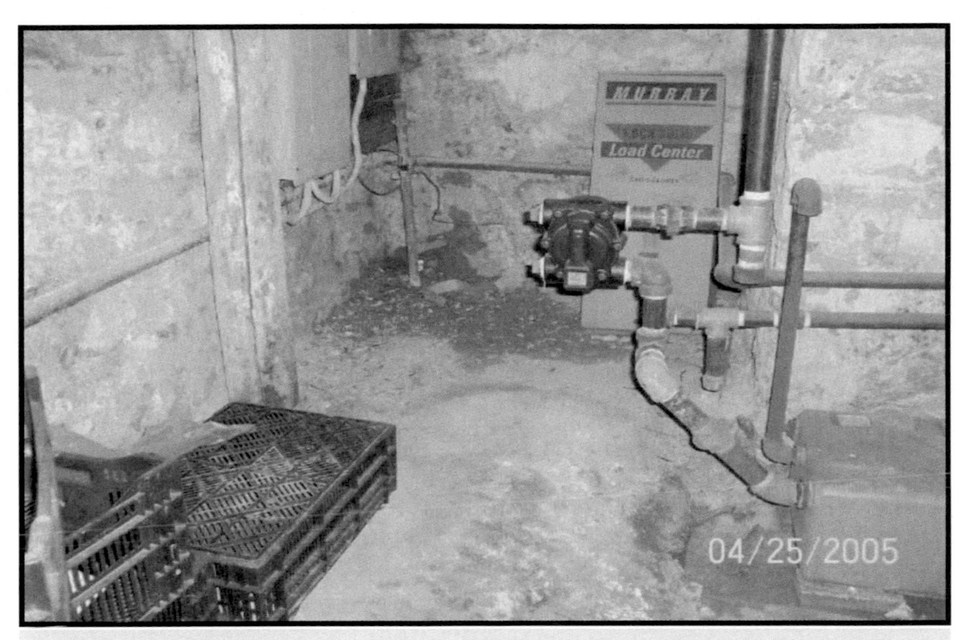

See the Appendix for ways to prevent mold problems in unfinished basements.

Salem Witches

In 1692, in Salem, Massachusetts, over a dozen people were hanged or stoned to death after being convicted of practicing witchcraft. Several were young girls who exhibited hallucinations and bizarre behaviors. Records show that part of their theology "examination" included being fed bread baked from rye flour and their urine. This test was supposed to help the spiritual authorities identify witches.

One toxic mold, called ergot, grows on rye and other grains. It contains a number of neurotoxic agents: the ergot alkaloids. Bread made from ergot-contaminated rye causes hallucinations. One of the most powerful ergot alkaloids is a derivative of lysergic acid (LSD). People who eat the contaminated rye would seem demon possessed when they are actually "stoned" on mold toxins. *Science* magazine recently reported new evidence[15] that the Salem witch trials followed an outbreak of rye ergot.

There are also other types of ergot (mold toxin) poisoning symptoms, e.g., gangrenous and convulsive. Both gangrenous and convulsive responses were found in Salem along with hallucinations and bizarre behavior.

People at Salem who contracted gangrenous ergotism suffered dry gangrene of the extremities. This caused their infected body parts to fall off.

Convulsive ergotism was epidemic in the Middle Ages and was known as *ignis sacer*, the holy fire. Sufferers of convulsive ergotism had crawling sensations in the skin, tingling in the fingers, vertigo, headaches, disturbances in sensation, painful muscular contractions, epileptic convulsions, and mania.

Every one of these convulsive symptoms appears in the records of the Salem witch trials. These symptoms are important because they link neurological symptoms to mold toxin exposure—in this case, ergot mold poisoning. Food poisoning from mold toxins is typically caused by a single type of mold. However, in a moldy building, we see a highly varied mix of mold toxins causing illness.

The Salem witch trials are historical evidence of mold toxin exposure causing symptoms that are much more serious than the typical runny nose and red eyes commonly attributed to mold toxins!

Treating a Farm Animal Better than Your Child

Scientists have long understood the dangers that toxic mold growing on wet grains has on both farm animals and farmers. An army of researchers at the U.S. Department of Agriculture work on "toxic mold." A search of the USDA Web site for "toxic" and "mold" garners 415 results. "Mold" brings up more than 1,000 results.

Efforts to protect livestock from mold toxins are underway worldwide. For instance, one Brazilian Department of Agriculture Web site, *www.micotoxinas.com.br*, lists graduate courses in Brazil on mycotoxin poisons.

All this talk about body and brain damage from indoor mold toxins might sound like the latest science fiction. But don't be fooled. There is plenty of recent history to back it up.

One of many toxic mold cases occurred about 75 years ago in Eastern Europe. Horses and other animals became seriously ill by a mysterious disease. Their symptoms included irritation of the mouth, throat and nose, damaged skin, excessive bleeding, nervous disorders, and death. In 1938, Russian scientists traced the disease to mold growing on the straw and grain fed to the affected animals.

Intensive studies followed. Researchers fed cultures of the fungus to healthy horses. Each horse ate servings of the fungus from Petri plates. Eating the contents of just one plate made them sick. Thirty of these small servings killed every one of these large animals.

These studies demonstrate the toxic nature of some molds. The mold in the horse study turned out to be *Stachybotrys* (Black mold). Since then, the toxic effects of *Stachybotrys* and many other molds have been found on numerous farms all over the world.

Most outbreaks of stachybotryotoxicosis were associated with stored wet hay or feed contaminated by *Stachybotrys*. As little as one milligram of toxin is reported to cause death in a huge horse. That is one ten-millionth of an ounce! A person merely touching or breathing in the presence of contaminated straw can develop toxic reactions. This is the same *Stachybotrys* found in many wet homes, schools and other structures.

T-2 or Tricothecene Sickness

Between the 1950s and the 1980s, reports on toxic mold started to appear more regularly, despite the complete lack of medical training about toxic molds that could help child and adult physicians "see" or diagnose mold illness. One report came out in 1986, when Dr. Croft[16] and his colleagues reported patients with trichothecene sickness—a mold toxin found in a Chicago home.

For five years, members of a Chicago family complained of headaches, sore throats, flu symptoms, recurring colds, diarrhea, fatigue, and general malaise. Mold was eventually discovered to be growing on moist debris in the home's hidden air ducts and on wood fiber ceiling material. It was detected in the air by standard air sampling procedures. The house had a chronic moisture problem that caused the mold growth.

Researchers tested extracts from the air duct debris and contaminated building materials and found they were toxic to test animals. They identified several mold toxins in addition to trichothecene. When the home's moisture and mold problems were corrected, the family's symptoms disappeared.

We now know that toxic mold can grow on all kinds of common modern building materials, such as fiberboard and drywall. But it can grow on paper, dust and lint as well. All it takes for toxic mold to grow is constant moisture from water damage, excessive humidity, water leaks, condensation, water infiltration, or flooding.

More than just "Black Mold" or *Stachybotrys*

In a 1998 report, Dr. Michael Hodgson[17] and fellow researchers describe a mold-contaminated courthouse and office building. What they described is a routine finding in old government structures with a history of leaks and excess moisture. But this building was brand new.

Almost immediately when they moved in, people in the courthouse developed fatigue, headaches, chest tightness, and pulmonary disease.

The defective building had serious moisture problems, and interior surfaces were heavily contaminated with *Aspergillus*, and *Penicillium* molds (and some *Stachybotrys*). Mold toxins from all three molds showed up in moldy ceiling tiles and on wallpaper.

Extensive Modern Day Medical Evidence.

There is extensive medical data showing that groups of sick people, when removed from sick buildings, either recovered on their own or with the help of Cholestyramine. At the same time, others that refused to leave the buildings got sicker.

Progressive medical mold treatments, such as Cholestyramine toxin-binding treatment, along with removal from the toxic environment, together can result in dramatic improvement, particularly if used promptly after the onset of mold toxin illness. When you see this happening over and over again, then these results become compelling evidence that links the toxic mold commonly found in water-damaged (sick) buildings to many types of illness.

CHAPTER 8

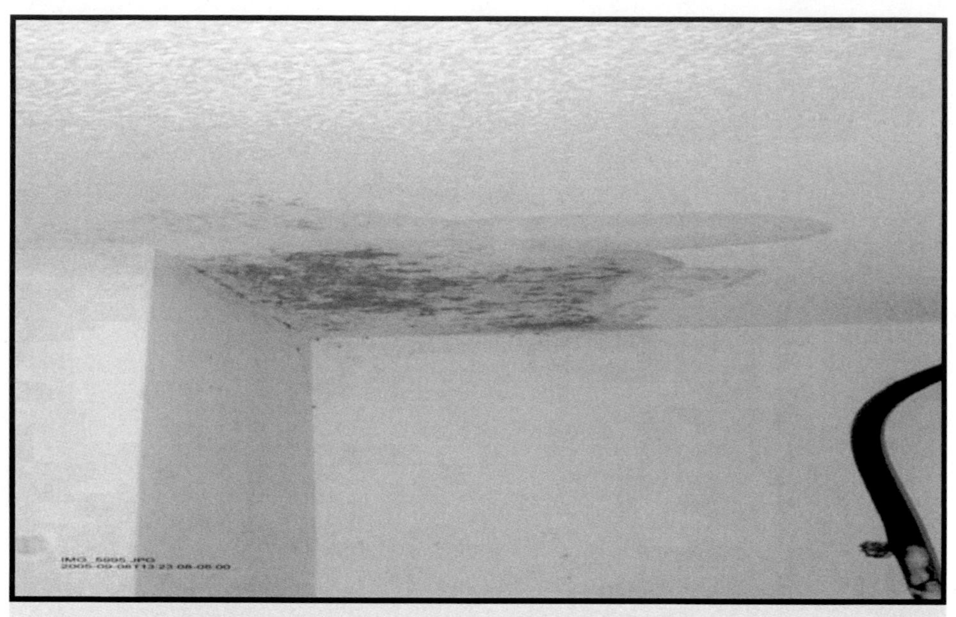

A tub overflowed in the 2nd story bedroom above this ceiling stain/mold growth. The mold growth inside the walls and ceiling was approximately 20 times the size of this visible problem.

Is Your Child or Grandchild in a Sick School?

Schools are far too casual about leaks and high humidity. When mold is found in a school, we hear excuses, rationalizations, finger pointing and buck-passing. It's the school district's problem, and they're notoriously under-funded. It's the federal government's fault for not providing more money or better guidelines. It's the building contractor cutting corners. It's the architects. They're not concerned or they just do not understand indoor air quality. It's the county or state building codes; they don't cover schools. Or there is no code enforcement.

The bottom line is that schools are the responsibility of each state. Lack of adequate state controls are making kids sick. It is time for state legislators to fix moldy schools and other state government buildings—not just moldy Governors' mansions.

School Buildings Must be Treated like Commercial or Residential High-Rises

Water damage causes mold. Mold releases toxins. If moisture damage or toxic mold turns up in a high-rise or other private building, the problem gets resolved ... fast.

When the developer of a new construction high-rise finds mold or moisture damage during or after construction, he makes the general contractor fix it.

If the contractor does not fix it, the developer fixes it by hiring someone else and bills the general contractor.

However, builders of defective schools are rarely held responsible.

In most states, building codes do not apply or are not enforced for school construction. Schools are state buildings and exempt from local county code enforcement.

New schools go up with no regard for healthy indoor air quality. Most school air conditioning systems cannot efficiently control indoor moisture in humid environments while simultaneously providing adequate fresh air.

Officials may claim they don't have the funds to properly build schools. But the problem lies in corruption. Here's how it works: the contractor bids on a school with a low cost, poor quality air conditioning system. This system is so inefficient and costly to run, that it cannot be cost effectively used to provide good indoor air quality. The outside air dampers that bring in fresh outside air are opened once, during the first (and usually last) inspection of the school's AC system upon completion of the school.

Once the inspectors leave, the outside air source is permanently sealed even though it is against building codes. The sealed rooms fill with moisture from roof and window leaks, wet clothes, and perspiring children. The trapped moisture promotes the growth of indoor mold.

Schools in Poor Countries Have a Secret

Kids with health problems due to toxic mold are generally found only in developed countries. Why? Because in developing countries, schools have a constant source of fresh outside air—open windows. These schools may have leaky roofs, poor construction, and toxic mold. *But the children are not sealed into rooms with mold toxins.* They breathe mostly fresh air. So, while they may feel pretty warm, they don't get sick from biotoxins at school.

Cheating On Our Kids' Health

Saving money with this AC system "trick" is happening hundreds and hundreds of times around the country. And why should the builders change their evil ways? After all, this is business. They don't care about your sick kids. (Their kids probably go to private schools anyway). And since school boards approve the school designs, contractors will not argue with cheap, junk AC systems being the rule of the land.

Solutions

☑ Award school contracts that consider the cost to properly operate an energy efficient, quality air conditioning system that controls indoor humidity, provides mandated fresh air levels, filters the air of impurities, and controls temperature (just like those that operate in new Federal office buildings or new first-class high-rise office buildings).

☑ Stop leaks early. Like cancer, if leaks are ignored and allowed to spread, the results can be catastrophic.

U.S. Schools vs. European Schools

In Europe, where funds for schools are also limited, there is a general consensus that indoor mold growth is toxic. European governments have wisely studied indoor air quality in schools. There, water-damaged schools are considered a health problem and fixing them is a very high priority. Here it is merely a nuisance when parents complain about mold in schools.

Powerful Lessons from Finland

Dr.Meklin[18] studied thirty-two Finnish school buildings, and over 5,000 students. She discovered that:

1. Due to the extreme cold in Finland, schools were not properly ventilated in order to save on energy costs. Poor ventilation contributes to moisture damage by increasing water condensation.
2. When a school's moisture damage and mold problems were addressed, kids returned to good health.
3. Schools with good ventilation and no moisture damage had very low instances of diseases related to indoor air quality.
4. School air pollution included bacteria, viruses, and toxic substances from deteriorating furnishings, carpets, and cleaning materials.
5. The highest disease-producing molds in Finnish schools were *Penicillium* and *Aspergillus.*

No study of this magnitude has been done in the United States due to limited government funding or interest.

Sample symptoms reported by Finnish school children in mold-contaminated schools included:

- Fatigue
- A 350% higher rate of asthma
- Respiratory infections
- Eye irritation

- Increased visits to physicians and use of antibiotics

Symptoms Finnish school personnel reported:

- Fatigue
- Headache
- Stuffy nose
- Eye irritation
- Nausea
- Sleeping difficulties

Again, this is yet another study—and there are too many with similar results to include them all—in which we see that categorizing mold toxin illness as merely a case of a runny nose and a little asthma is simply to deny a huge base of quality scientific and medical evidence.

CHAPTER 9

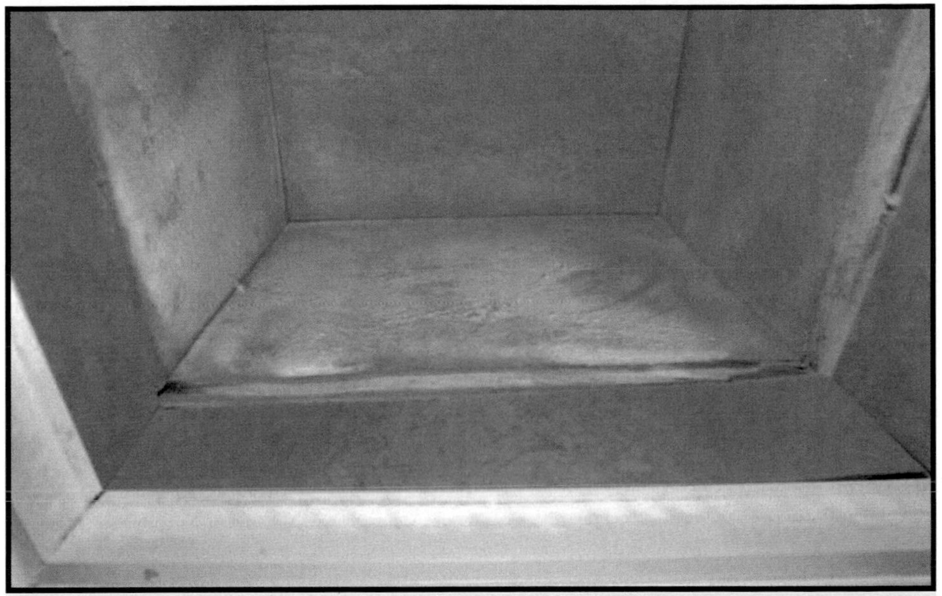

Mold-covered dust is caked on the inside of this air duct because no air filter was used. The entire house smelled of mold due to contaminated air ducts. The answer is not trying to clean fragile AC ducts; rather, it is using good air filters and CHANGING THEM OFTEN. This way, the ducts don't get dirty in the first place.

Tools to Fix Your Child's Situation

There is no simple pill that will always fix your child's situation. "Treatment" may involve everything from filing various types of insurance claims, to using special air filters, to cleaning and storing important items. We discuss these helpful options and others below. Certainly, a first key treatment is a reduction in toxin exposure. Removing mold can be as easy as squirting bleach on a small patch of mold growing in a bedroom corner. But it can be "difficult" when the mold contamination is so extensive that the homeowner cannot easily afford to have the work done properly.

Mold is a result of excess humidity and/or water damage. In most cases when the problems are very extensive in homes, the remediation will be covered by home owners insurance or a builder's liability "construction defect" policy. But in most cases, the insurance company or builder will initially deny your claim. You will have to persist and may need an attorney to help you. Here are some basics that you need to understand to help you recover.

Builder's Liability

Most serious water related problems—including air conditioner contamination—in newer homes are the result of construction defects. If these building errors cause you or your children to become ill, the home warranties do not expire in the common warranty time of 1-2 years. In most states the builder remains responsible for a minimum of 12 years for water damage from a building error. Furthermore, you do not have to be the original owner of the house to hold the builder accountable. In other states, hidden defects are covered for 2-3 years after discovery.

So in almost all cases, you should look to the builder to fix defects that result in water damage and mold in newer homes.

A number of the major builders will automatically handle all water-related claims regardless of the warranty period. But most builders need to be forced to do so.

Once the builder agrees to fix the problem, they will want to use their own people. The problem is, their own people don't know anything about mold. They will more than likely contaminate your home when they remove the moldy materials.

Every subcontractor that the builder employs will have a substantial insurance policy for the work that is required. You should demand the same. Demand that the mold work be done by a company that is insured for at least $1 million in mold coverage.

And demand that the builder provide you with a certificate that the remediated home is now mold free—that is, as good as new. More than likely they will not agree to do this, but will ask you to find someone that meets your needs. So go ahead and hire a qualified consultant to do the work. You can then have your cake and eat it too.

Locating a Local Lawyer

Quite often, nothing will get done unless you have an attorney's help. The key to getting the right lawyer is to have good documentation of the mold problem. Make sure that you have plenty of pictures of really ugly-looking mold. If the mold is hidden inside a wall, then you will need to have someone open that wall and take pictures of ugly mold. Builders know that if those pictures are shown to a jury, they are dead meat. Make sure you have a qualified person doing the testing and construction defect report for you. Rarely will an attorney take this sort of work on a contingency basis. Be prepared to spend some money.

Your Local Doc

If positive, lab results can show that mold is making you or your child sick. Add those to the mold testing results and pictures of the mold in your home. It also would be useful to have people who have witnessed any new mold illness or symptoms write a note explaining their observations. If eight people write a two-paragraph note saying that once your child moved into the moldy home they suddenly lost functioning, you would have some pretty powerful testimony. These notarized notes can be put in the medical file. Your attorney will know what to do with this medical material.

Air Filters in Schools

Demand that school officials put your child in a clean classroom. However, it is entirely possible that no classroom in the school is mold free. But, if you can get the school to put high quality "MERV 11" HEPA filters in the main AC system, you will have helped immensely. If not, then see if you can bring an air filtration machine into the classroom. You will probably need a few. Do not use any air purifiers that produce toxic ozone.

The table below shows that the "junky," blue, see-through fiberglass filters and the low-cost pleated (MERV 7) filters do not filter out any of the very small particles, including allergens and mold spores. It also shows that a MERV 11 filter is about twice as efficient in filtering out these small particles as a MERV 9 filter.

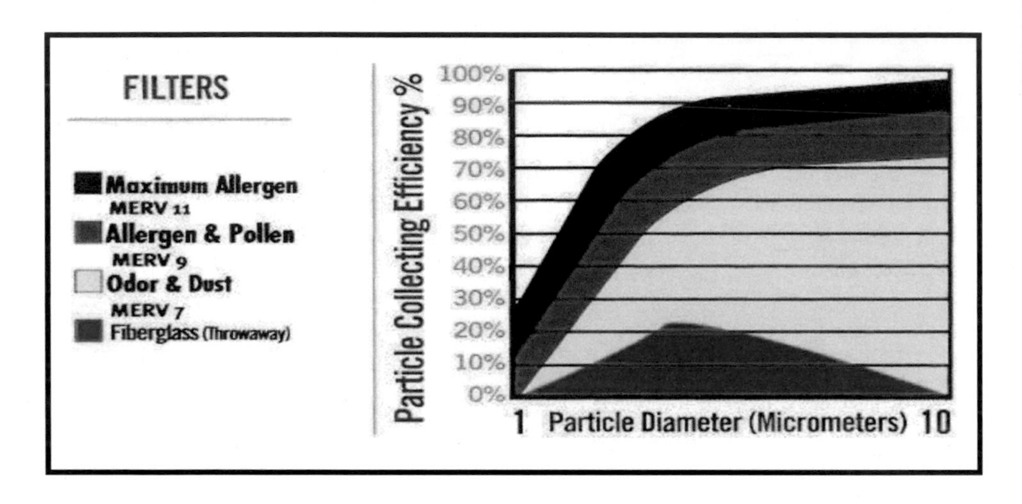

Do-it-Yourself Air Purifier for Homes or Schools

Actually a $15, 20-inch box fan with a 20-inch MERV 11 HEPA filter taped to the back works very well. Two of these in a classroom or sick child's room will have everyone breathing easier in about two days. Change the filters once a month so they do not lose effectiveness.

Controlling Indoor Humidity

As long as there are no water leaks, controlling indoor humidity so that it is below 65% will prevent mold from growing in a residence or office. When the indoor humidity is low, even a small leak usually will not result in mold if the water dries quickly.

Levels of indoor bacteria, viruses, respiratory infections, and dust mites are also significantly reduced when indoor humidity levels are controlled.

The chart on the following page, published by the Australian Government, shows that mold growth, bacterial, dust mites and viruses are virtually eliminated when the indoor humidity is kept between 30% and 55%. Since 40% humidity is uncomfortable for people, the ideal range is 40%-55%.

OPTIMUM INDOOR RELATIVE HUMIDITY & AIR QUALITY GUIDE

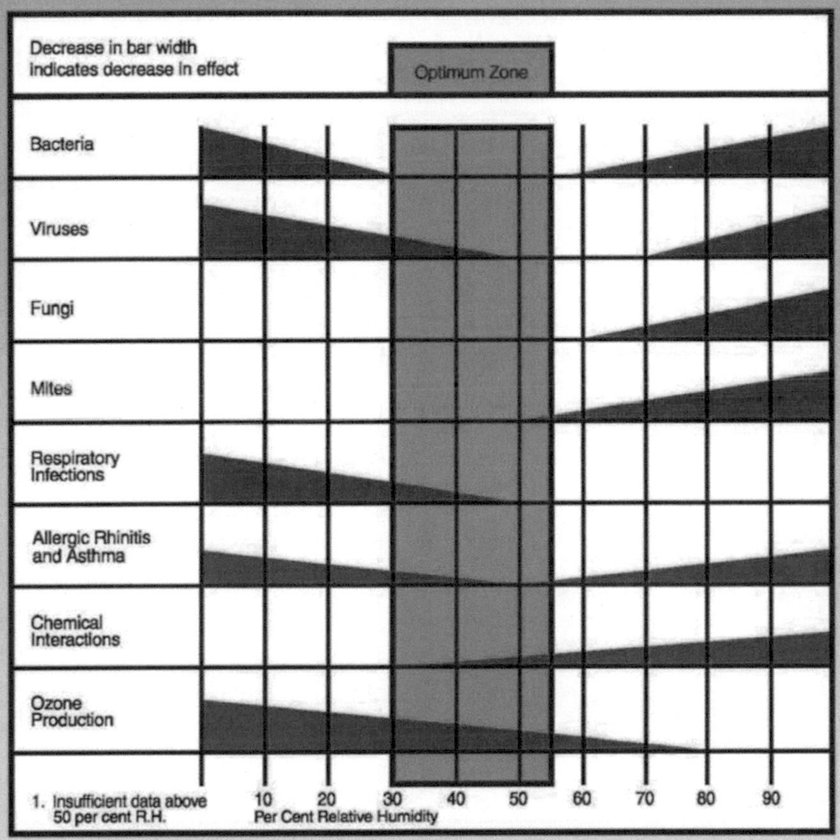

(Source - Theodore D. Sterling and Associates, Canada)

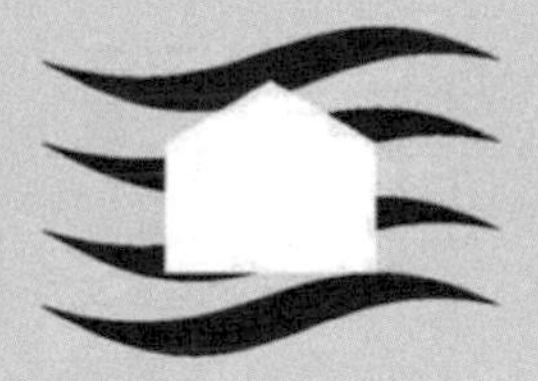

Controlling indoor humidity levels is item #5 on the EPA's list of **Ten Things You Should Know About Mold** (*www.epa.gov/mold/moldresources.html*):

> *Reduce indoor humidity to decrease mold growth by: venting bathrooms, dryers, and other moisture-generating sources to the outside; using air conditioners and de-humidifiers; increasing ventilation; and using exhaust fans whenever cooking, dishwashing and cleaning.*

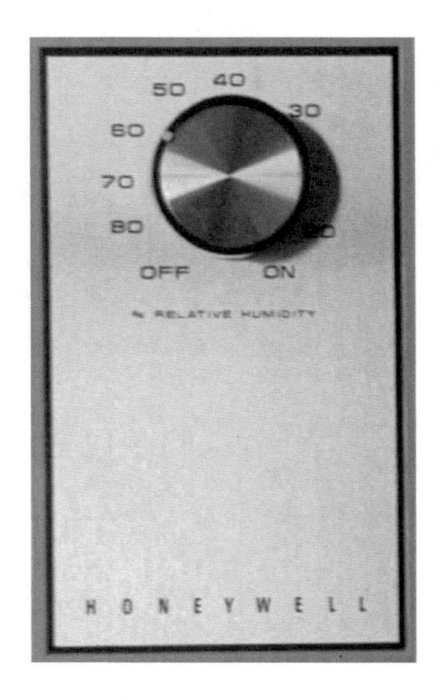

Using an existing AC system, people can accurately control their indoor humidity by installing a low-cost humidistat that is connected to the AC thermostat. The AC is then controlled both by humidity levels and temperature. If the humidity rises above the target level, typically 60%, the AC is turned on and runs until the humidity drops below 60%. Of course, the thermostat also still works and turns the AC on when the temperature rises above the set level.

The most popular humidistat is the Honeywell H46C 1000 Humidistat (pictured at left), which is about $50 at Home Depot. It takes an electrician about only 10 minutes to install.

Mold Remediation: Cleaning Mold from Your Home

It is important to understand that visible mold is more of a problem to people's health than mold sealed inside of walls. The first thing to do when people are sick is to eliminate the water source so that mold growth stops; then eliminate all visible mold. Mold spores become airborne when disturbed so be careful not to disturb mold. Never brush or sweep mold or direct a fan or AC duct toward mold growth.

Before starting mold clean up, always have a fan in a window pointed out during any work so released mold spores generally end up outside and not in your house. And you should always wear an N-95 face mask that you can buy for about $2.50 from Home Depot or Wal-Mart. These are not the painter's masks that sell for 99 cents. Make sure the mask says N-95 on the package. The N-95 mask protects against mold spores but not the fumes from the straight bleach you will use to clean mold. If you are sensitive to bleach smells, have someone else do the mold cleaning. Wear eye protection, such as goggles, and proper gloves when working with bleach.

Cleaning Procedure

1. Close the door to the room. Open a window in the problem room and put a fan in the window sill pointing out. Turn the fan on MAX. This will suck out any loose mold spores released during your mold-cleaning activities.
2. Wearing gloves, goggles and your N-95 mask, put straight bleach on 2-3 folded-up paper towels and dampen any mold spots on the ceiling, walls, baseboards, or cabinets. Make sure you protect the carpet.
3. Discard paper towels when they become "dirty" with mold. Do not carry them through the house. Place them into a plastic bag and discard. Use fresh paper towels as often as needed until the job is done.
4. Repeat after 30 minutes as needed.
5. Seal any openings in walls or ceilings with plaster, duct tape, or expanding foam. Using tape or caulking, seal not only any cracks or openings in the walls or ceilings, but also all electrical plates, baseboards, and other openings.

Cleaning Your Home after Mold Remediation

If used alone, even MERV 11 air filters on your AC system are not sufficient to clean your moldy home. They will start to clean the air, but if the house has mold-contaminated dust on the floors, furniture, or other contents, then as fast as the filters remove the mold contaminants from the air, new contaminants will be re-suspended into the air from contaminated dust.

To properly clean a house that has had mold problems, all of the settled dust must be removed. Never dust with a duster!

Wipe surfaces with paper towels sprayed with a dust magnet. And make sure your vacuum cleaner is equipped with an allergen-type HEPA filter bag. If they do not make one for your model, buy a new vacuum—unless you want to blow billions of mold and toxin-covered dust particles all over a room as you "clean."

Before attempting to clean settled dust, you will need to equip your AC system with a MERV 11 filter and have the FAN turned ON. Plus, you should put a few Do-It-Yourself Air Purifiers in each room as you clean. This will prevent you from dispersing mold spores and mold-contaminated dust all over your home. (See Chapter 14 for details on air conditioning and air filter issues.)

Fabric furniture must be thoroughly HEPA vacuumed, and drapes should be HEPA vacuumed or dry cleaned.

Again, all dust in the house must be removed. This means the tops of fan blades, window sills, art frames and plants must be cleaned. All the furniture and appliances need to be moved to access hidden areas for cleaning. When the cleaning is finished, check for dust by wiping with a clean white cloth. Clean again, if necessary, until there is no more settled dust.

If the house was contaminated by *Stachybotrys*, we recommend that you do even more thorough cleaning to remove *Stachybotrys* biotoxins from the home and contents. This will include steam vacuum cleaning all furniture, carpets and drapes with the new SteamVacs that clean with both steam and detergent-based cleaning agents. We personally use the Hoover Agility model, but many other models should work well.

Removing Moldy Carpet

1. Place a $15.00 box fan in an open window blowing OUT.
2. Close the doors to the room and turn off the room's HVAC (AC, Ventilation, and Heating System).

3. Vacuum the carpet with a HEPA vacuum or a vacuum equipped with special allergen HEPA bag.
4. Lightly mist the entire carpet with water, Lysol or another household cleaner.
5. Cut the carpet into 3-4 pieces with a new sharp carpet tool.
6. Roll up the carpet with the back of the carpet on the outside.
7. Do not carry the carpet through the home! Push it through an open window.
8. If you need to carry it through your home, seal it in 3-6 mil plastic first. If there are any possible leaks, seal it again. Seal the plastic with duct tape.
9. Take the carpet to the dump in the bed of a truck. Do not transport it inside your car or van unless it is completely sealed twice in plastic wrap.

Keys to Properly Storing Contents

Contents stored in basements or attics routinely become moldy. One of the keys to saving paper or wood-based materials is understanding that moisture or humidity can damage them. Also, avoid hot and cold extremes so items do not become brittle.

Moisture will dissolve, stain, mildew, or mold your treasures.

Tip: Plastic tubs with a tight seal can keep many artifacts safe from water and mold. They also protect against air pollution, insects and rodents. If you will be storing paper or wood protects in plastic tubs for long periods of time, lightly spray Lysol (alcohol-based) disinfectant on the contents, let them dry, and then seal them in the tubs. Do not spray any valuable artifacts that might be damaged by alcohol.

CHAPTER 10

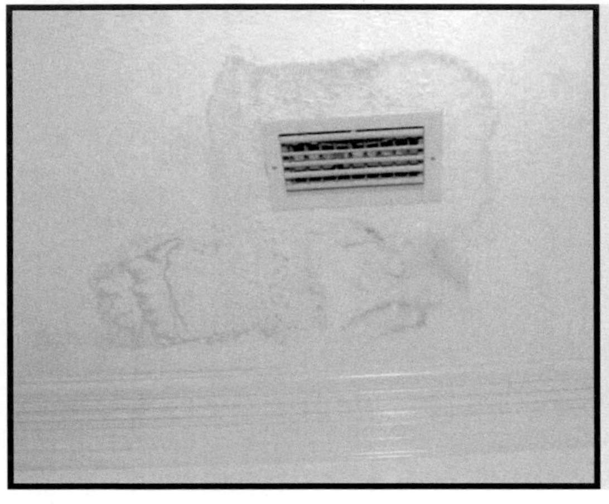

When we looked inside the attic, we determined that this mold problem was not from the AC system, but rather, a roof leak. The roof leak just happened to be on top of the AC supply duct. Amazingly, the homeowners had ignored this mold growth in the master bedroom closet for 2 years! Since the husband traveled, he was not exposed as often. But the wife was so sick she could not get out of bed. Neither suspected that the she was ill from mold.

Decreased Insight: A *Deadly* Mold Symptom

"Their brain is too mold fogged. They will never get it!"

"Why call them 'hopeless?'" I asked.

Shaking his head, John said, "Doc, many people are so affected by long term exposure to toxic mold that it has massively affected their ability to think," The veteran mold remediator added, "You will never see these people, Doc, because they do not feel they have a problem. They are too far gone. Once the mold affects them, they lose the ability to see themselves realistically. They are moody, restless, foggy, and forgetful. If they are talented or brilliant, they may still be able to function, but not at their true potential."

Doctor Duh

Many years ago, I (Schaller) lived in a lovely old home with many leaks but a great deal of charm. The magnificent home had huge rooms and very high ceilings. My research books and papers were stacked from the floor to the ceiling. The small amount of visible mold on the baseboards and behind furniture never caught my attention. I liked all of my books, but so did my "mold roommates."

My "roommates" arrived with the first roof and window leaks many years ago, and they never left. The landlord explained about the leaks, "In a big old house, you never can be sure you closed up all the openings."

About nine months after I moved into the lovely, old, moldy home I started becoming moody and gaining weight. I gained it very slowly. I figured age had caught up with me, but I was not that old. Soon I was overweight. At night I would lie in bed and look up at the stars through my massive old windows, and ask, "Why am I gaining all this weight?" As I looked up at the water stains on the high ceilings, it never occurred to me that what I thought were small crack lines were actually thin threads of visible mold. Only after working as the second author on *Mold Warriors* did I understand what had happened. I had gained the weight and become moody due to mold in my house. Now, every week, I see the same thing happening with my patients.

Mold toxins can make geniuses blind to their problems. They undermine the front part of the brain, which is involved in self-awareness. Bluntly, you have "egg on your face," and don't even know it.

Child and Parent Insight

Fixing the problem with your child can be hindered by frontal lobe trouble. And guess who can have impaired insight? It can be both your child and all the adults involved. The parents can be exposed to home mold and have poor insight, while teachers and administrators at your child's school can be exposed to the same school mold. Therefore, they can have reduced insight into the cause of their own illness, not to mention your child's.

*****

Amy's son has "ADHD." It started when he was twelve, which is ridiculous—you do not suddenly get impulsive and unfocussed at twelve. Amy's family moved into a lovely California home eight months ago. She said they had no mold. "Not a chance! Please, there is just no way we have mold in our home!" After I ruled out about a hundred other possibilities, I begged her to do an air sample. She told me I was "a terrible listener" and that I was "wasting her money." Her home air sample results showed that her mold problem was hidden and serious. After $4,500.00 in mold remediation repairs, paid for by her builder's insurance, her son's "ADHD" slowly vanished over five months. And her mild postnasal drip and fogginess were gone in a month. "I cannot believe that I did not notice these symptoms in myself," she said. Amy had poor insight caused by mold toxins.

*****

"Dr. Schaller, my childhood school was an old leaky building and I was never sick from mold. Your mold concern seems like a fad to me," Dr. Hendricks said. He was the Dean of a respected private school in New England. I had just met two siblings from his school, who flew in to see me. Both were having mood and anxiety symptoms, and their parents wanted another opinion.

Both children also had "auditory processing problems." I ruled out other illnesses including Lyme and Bartonella, and finally asked about their school. The siblings, Daniel and Lynn, spoke very casually about the leaks in their school. They mentioned that my "mold picture book" looked like their school. They were clueless and had no insight into the leaks or mold being related to their troubles. Mold toxins had made them tired, bored and emotionally flat.

I told their parents that to help determine if mold was a cause of their children's problems, some basic mold testing of the school should be performed. The Dean explained to the father that they had done mold testing in February of the previous year, and the results were "negative." Thankfully, the parents had donated a little money to the school, and the school did not want to simply blow them off.

Also, when I explained that the air samples were going to be done for free, Dean Hendricks seemed to tolerate the idea. I am sure he thought, "Hey, if you want to waste time and money second guessing our past consultant, I will not stop you." To his credit, he did not stonewall the testing out of fear of accountability.

When the new round of sampling came back strongly positive for mold, the parents offered to have a leading mold investigator fly in to do further testing. Nine locations were found that had toxin-forming mold and some toxin-forming bacteria. The "sick" moldy locations included areas near Daniel, Lynn and a teacher who had complained the previous year—she had been the catalyst for the earlier testing.

The Dean and the Board made the necessary building repairs, and after a year of medical treatment, both siblings are now off all medications and doing well.

Amazingly, neither the Dean nor the siblings still really accept that mold was the cause of their problems. The Dean merely says, "We were happy to make the changes that were required." But he is annoyed he had to pay for the modest remediation work.

Mold illness can blind you.

Following the remediation and medical treatment, the siblings returned to their normal behavior. They are able to reach out, make friends, study, and have a better mood because they no longer have toxic mold inflammation in their body! Yet they credit their new success at school to "nicer teachers" and a year of "medication." They still do not get it!

CHAPTER 11

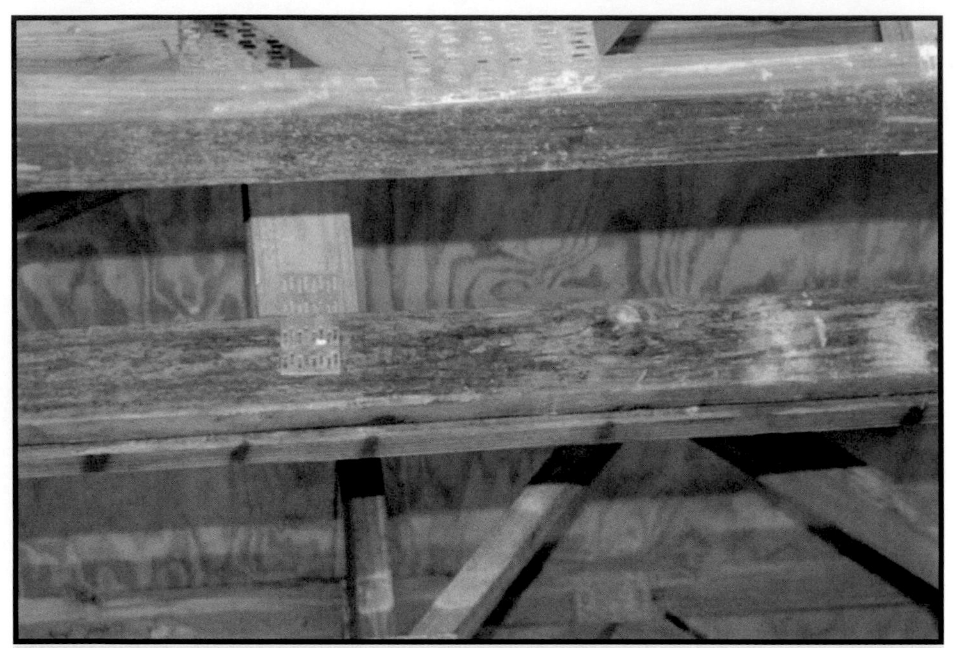

Moldy wood trusses in a new house under construction. You don't want your kids playing in this attic!

How Biotoxins Affect Vision

Mold toxins often cause subtle changes in vision that you cannot easily notice. The Visual Contrast Sensitivity Test (VCST) is an easy and inexpensive mold toxin exposure test offered over the Internet.

The Visual Contrast Sensitivity Test (VCST)

This special test is not done during eye exams with eye doctors. It does not test vision. It tests inflammation and toxin exposure in the brain. To understand how it works, you need to understand how the eye nerves work. Simply put, the eye nerves divide up on their way to the back of your head where images are "read." Each eye nerve goes through both sides of the brain, and along the top and bottom of the brain.

So guess what happens if the brain is exposed to a biotoxin? You may still be able to see 20/20, but you will have errors on this special visual contrast test. The "contrast" part is the key to it. The test involves looking at light and dark grey lines that have different degrees of contrast and width, and picking the direction that the lines point.

In a biotoxin-exposed brain, the ability to distinguish the direction of these tiny light and dark grey lines is diminished.

You can purchase these tests in sets of three at *www.chronicneurotoxins.com*.

The VCST is not specific to mold illness. It shows very subtle problems from many causes. Some brief examples would be:

- Petroleum toxins or other solvent exposures
- Lyme, Babesia, or other common tick-borne toxin-producing infections
- Toxins from various dangerous algae
- Diabetes
- Parkinson's
- Alzheimer's

So perhaps the best way to view this test is as an option for seeing subtle but serious effects of biological toxins, foreign chemicals, or inflammation that may be easily missed by the patients and doctors. If you get a positive result, you are quite ill, but may not know it. On the other hand, you can be ill from mold toxins even if the VCST does not detect it.

While a manual VCST is a little more accurate, you also can order a computer screen VCST at *http://www.chronicneurotoxins.com/registration/index.cfm*. The computer screen test can be useful for quickly and inexpensively tracking improvement or relapse.

CHAPTER 12

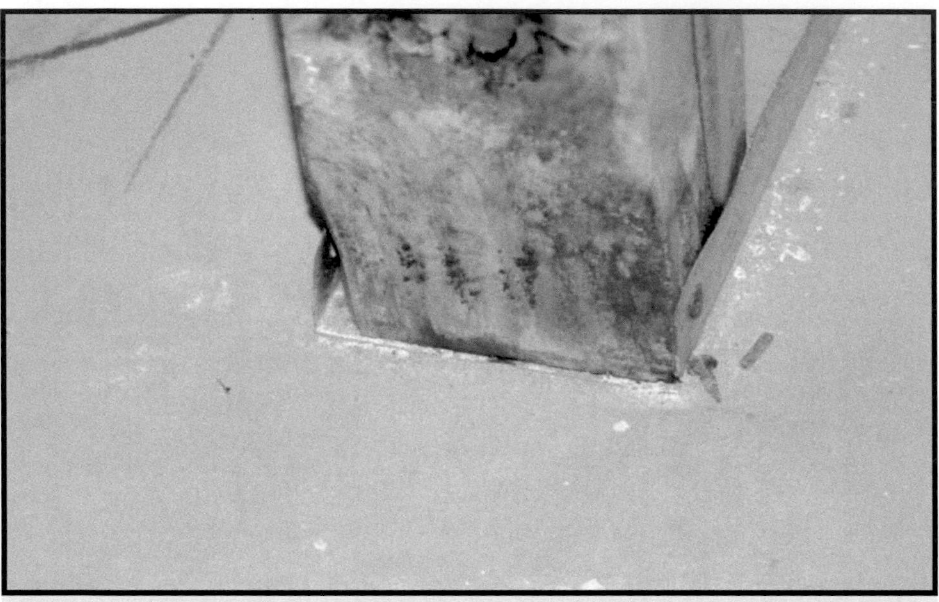

Here's a moldy 2x4 in the door frame of a new house under construction. We recommend that home buyers inspect homes under construction for mold problems like this.

Medical Mold Treatment

There are four common errors with medical treatment for Sick Building Syndrome exposure.

☑ The first error is not considering that mold biotoxins could be the problem. Mold biotoxins reduce insight, causing medical care to be neglected.

☑ Next, during treatment, people continue to get exposed to the toxins at the same (or even another) sick school, home or office. You can't fix the body if it continues being exposed to high levels of biotoxins. If you plan on cutting corners regarding exposure, then simply plan on staying ill.

☑ If the problem was in a home and it was remediated, 100% of the indoor contaminated dust must be removed. Even after treatment, a person will be highly sensitive to mold biotoxin exposure for some time. So, the entire home and contents must be brought to "like new" condition.

☑ Finally, many feel if they remediate the problem building, all the problems with their body will fall back into place. For some this is true. But for many, problems with biotoxin exposure do not reverse without a number of special treatments. Thankfully, many of these treatments are covered by insurance.

An Accidental Discovery

One critical treatment for mold biotoxin cleansing comes as a result of investigations from a Maryland lakes disaster. Fish were dying in huge numbers and many people were getting ill.

One day as dozens of these folks were filling Dr. Ritchie Shoemaker's Maryland office, he gave a woman an older medication that stops diarrhea: Cholestyramine. At her next appointment, not only was her diarrhea gone, but many of her other body and brain symptoms went away. Since then, Dr. Shoemaker has used Cholestyramine on thousands of patients and finds it very good at binding a specific type of toxins—biotoxins.

Detoxification with Cholestyramine: Options and Solutions (Advice for Medical Professionals)

The cheapest form of Cholestyramine (CSM) has been available for over twenty years, and is covered by most insurance plans. It comes in packets sweetened with regular sugar or aspartame ("Lite"). Adults with significant toxin exposure typically take at least four packets a day.

Ideal Child Dose Varies

Many factors determine the best dose, including intensity of past mold exposure, ongoing mold exposure, MSH blood level, and a youth's ability to function. We generally give pre-adolescents or youth under seventy pounds one packet per day. Adolescents typically take two packets if their MSH is normal and their home or school has no serious mold. If their MSH is under 35 or they have constant mold exposure, the recommendation is three packets a day. Since Cholestyramine (CSM) binds fat-soluble vitamins, we recommend a very good multivitamin. The highest quality wholesale nutrient we use with youth is NSI Prenatal which can be found on my (Schaller) website, *www.personalconsult.com.*

Some parents find it difficult to give Cholestyramine (CSM) to their children because some package inserts say it must be given 4 hours from food, but this is not necessary—1 hour is fine. If CSM is eaten too close to a meal, the CSM potency will be somewhat diminished since some food fat will be bound and excreted instead of toxins. The real issue with CSM dosing is to keep it from binding to your prescription medications. Therefore, when it comes to medication, we like patients to take Cholestyramine at least forty-five minutes away from medications (or fat-soluble vitamins). If it is an essential medication, keep it 90 minutes away from a dose of CSM (and discuss this with your health care provider).

Some youth do not like the taste of the mixed powder. However, they might take it if it is put in something other than water, such as orange juice, soda, tea, or skim milk. Children should be rewarded for their good medical compliance.

Capsule form of CSM

Capsules can be made into any size, but generally we use 300 mg capsules of CSM resin for small children, and 400 mg capsules for larger children. Some adults prefer larger 600 mg or even 800 mg capsules. These capsules have no sugar, no food coloring, and no fillers. However, patients needs to take about 6-8 capsules per dose to equal one packet. Also, many insurance companies do not cover the cost of these prescription compounded forms. So if you want them paid for, plan on a fight with your insurance carrier. One location to purchase CSM capsules, with a prescription, is Lionville Natural Pharmacy in Pennsylvania at 877-363-7474. They can ship all over the world. Other compounding pharmacists can also provide this service.

If a person has trouble with constipation with any form of CSM, we recommend adding minerals to the diet. That often helps. Many youth do well with a tablet of Zinc (L-Opti-Zinc) or some magnesium oxide added to their CSM. If the youth has pellet-like stools, they are constipated and this can result in hemorrhoids. They can use more Zinc and magnesium. If that fails, consider a half of a teaspoon of magnesium citrate morning and night. Magnesium citrate is used in very high doses to empty the entire thirty-foot bowel, so it always can stop constipation. If diarrhea develops, drop or decrease your magnesium citrate dose.

Some patients experience nausea or indigestion from the Cholestyramine. Sometimes this goes away in weeks. Any past or current exposure to mold toxins can also make the stomach sensitive. Some options for nausea from CSM include using Carafate to coat an irritated stomach, or an acid blocker like Pepsid. The latter may make some stomach enzymes less effective for digestion, but you might not have a choice. Some adults use enteric coated digestive enzymes that open after the stomach, but many children do not want more pills.

Many patients have been through several rounds of antibiotics and have their gut flora stripped. As a result they can have serious "indigestion." Such patients should take probiotics, or good bacteria, which are required for proper intestinal health. Types with good adherence to the intestinal wall are from Therabiotics, Natren, and Metagenics.

Other Mold Binders

Welchol is not as strong a binder as CSM, but some feel it helps them in high doses. It is available in pill form with a prescription. Activated Charcoal is used to bind many different drugs and toxins, but might not bind as well as CSM to some mold biotoxins. Some feel the fat binder Chitosan can bind mold toxins, and a few studies seem to show potential. However, mold medical experts currently do not use this. The benefits of Chitosan are that it is inexpensive, comes in pill form, and doesn't require a prescription.

Exercise Therapy

If you feel severe fatigue and muscle pain the next day after a work out, it may mean you have a VEGF abnormality. Decrease your exercise intensity and take at least nine Omega-3 capsules per day.

Inflammation

A diabetes medication, Actos, has been found to have strong anti-inflammation abilities. It is used by some mold experts to help "turn off" inflammation. However, some things must be understood before using. A child or adult cannot be in an active mold location, or the "turned off" genes will turn on again with mold toxin exposure. Also, we do not have much experience with the use of Actos in kids. Most doctors are too afraid of being sued for an "off label" use, and would be hard to convince to use it. If it is used, the youth probably should be willing to do arm blood testing. Arm blood testing is a new technology and, when done correctly, is absolutely painless and not at all like painful finger sticks. Any nurse practitioner, diabetes educator or nurse should be able to show you how to use a blood sugar arm tester. We have tried it on many patients with no complaints. Often patients ask when the testing is going to start—it is already done!

Actos is not a long-term medication for inflammation. It should be used for 3-4 weeks and then stopped for about 2 weeks to rest the liver. The dose should be started at 7.5-15 mg for a few days and then increased slowly to a maximum dose of 45 mg. The maximum dose for children and adolescents is not yet known. Furthermore, Actos requires a special no-amylose diet written about by Dr. Ritchie Shoemaker.

The diet is believed to reduce inflammation alone, though even more so with Actos. The toughest part of the diet is stopping grains and flours. You cannot have pasta, rice, wheat, oats or breads, or any type of flour. But you can have corn. Corn comes in many forms: corn flour, corn pastas, corn tortillas, and corn chips. But if amylase is added to a corn product, you cannot have it.

The good news is that you can eat all proteins and all vegetables except peanuts, beets, carrots and potatoes—no vegetables that grow in the ground. Plus, you can eat all fruits except bananas.

However, you should avoid all corn syrup and reduce your sugar intake. Many progressive health care providers have found that when the three pounds of good bacteria in your intestines are replaced with dangerous bacteria or yeast, your health is undermined. Limiting these sugars will help prevent the overgrowth of yeast in the intestinal tract.

For more details, see *www.moldwarriors.com*.

Abnormal VEGF Treatment

In our lab chapter, we explain that this hormone opens up and builds capillaries to allow good blood flow to reach the tissues. If it is abnormal, fatigue and cramping can develop, especially after exercise. One treatment is a very high dose of Omega-3 oils. These oils are becoming popular for good reasons. If you buy them, avoid some common errors. Think twice about buying flax oil or borage oil since these can have Omega-6 and -9 oils and these can be pro-inflammatory!

If your child is picky, but likes orange custard, consider trying Coromega. And if either you or your child has a sensitive stomach, some Omega-3 brands are enterically coated, which prevents the capsules from causing stomach indigestion. Metagenics offers a new brand of enterically-coated Omega-3 in large, potent capsules. Fisol, a smaller, enterically-coated capsule, is available at published wholesale prices from Vitacost (*www.vitacost.com*). Vitacost also sells a wide range of other Omega-3 products, including brands with small capsule sizes and various flavors.

Brain Fog

Removal from moldy places along with treatment with CSM can often stop brain fog. Another option is the use of Trental. It slightly lowers inflammation, but is useful in increasing blood flow to help lower brain fog. Some progressive physicians also suggest standardized *ginko biloba* for improved cognition, but the FDA does not support this health claim.

Autoimmunity Treatments

Inflammation can be invisible like high blood pressure or it can cause aching joints, swelling, bloating, headaches, and mood swings.

Inflammation can be severe enough to promote autoimmunity. Autoimmunity is usually found by blood test abnormalities showing that mold biotoxins have increased various parts of your inflammation response system, making it too aggressive. Instead of just attacking invading bacteria, your body is now attacking your own nerves, nerve fat, cell wall fat, and other body parts.

Inflammation and autoimmunity can be treated with magnesium, a mineral required in over 200 body reactions. Sublingual magnesium at 50-100 mg per day absorbed directly into the blood stream can help reduce not only inflammation and autoimmunity, but also high blood pressure, muscle aches, and spasms. Doses over 100 mg per day—delivered in minutes under the tongue—generally should not be used, as very large doses can cause low blood pressure. Using magnesium at higher doses can help treat mold-induced migraines, but you will need to monitor your blood pressure.

Sublingual lozenges only can be made by an experienced compounding pharmacist, such as the pharmacists at the Professional Compounding Centers of America (PCCA) in Houston, Texas. You can call them at 800-331-2498. If the sublingual magnesium options are hard to administer to your child, these pharmacists can also make a transdermal magnesium cream. The cream has approximately 20% absorption and is usually placed under some type of hypo-allergenic tape or wrap.

Steroids like prednisone or dexamethasone are another treatment option, but since these lower MSH, they only should be used sparingly and briefly, if at all.

Throughout the world, herbs are routinely used to decrease inflammation. Since traditional American physicians are closely tied to the pharmaceutical industry, they have little understanding of herbal treatments. Meanwhile, many progressive physicians believe herbs, such as nettle and curcumin, can decrease inflammation.[19,20] Some physicians also suggest taking a baby 81 mg enterically-coated aspirin.

Gliadin, a potentially troublesome part of wheat, can bother and inflame the intestines of some sensitive people. If the gut becomes inflamed from certain foods like wheat, stop eating wheat. Consider eating rice or corn products instead of wheat if you have symptoms or high gliadin antibodies on your lab results. Currently, it is getting easier to decrease wheat, since you can now get rice noodles, corn pasta, and even potato bagels.

Abnormal Urination

If a youth has excess urination and a lab result showing a very low anti-diuretic hormone (ADH), consider using DDAVP, a common bed-wetting medication prescribed by child psychiatrists and pediatricians.

Traditional Asthma & Allergy Treatments

The focus of this book is on the ability of mold biotoxins to hurt the entire body, not just the nose and lungs. Yet, mold can bother both the nasal areas and the lungs. Therefore, while allergy shots, antihistamines, nasal irrigation, and inhalers are not the primary treatments for mold toxins, they might help alleviate some allergy symptoms. These treatments should only supplement a broader mold toxin treatment program–they should not be the sole treatment.

Hormone Replacement Issues

Sometimes mold toxins disrupt the optimal functioning of both adult and adolescent hormones. The replacement of hormones with bio-identical options in adults and adolescents is a debated topic in some academic circles. Dr. Schaller has published a report in the world's largest pediatric journal on the successful use of natural progesterone transdermal cream in adolescents with PMS. His father, an IVY-league-trained OB/GYN, was prescribing some natural bio-identical hormones forty-five years ago. Of course, many patients already have weighed in on the debate by routinely using these natural hormones and buying books that support their use.

Pharmaceutical companies generally only support the use of synthetic, patented hormones and birth control pills. If you want to test for abnormal hormones from either aging or mold toxins, you need a health practitioner who will test for thyroid autoantibodies and a very wide range of hormones, including free testosterone, DHT, estradiol, progesterone, cortisol, free T3 thyroid, and free T4 thyroid. These should be tested in addition to hormones associated with mold illness, such as VIP, MSH and VEGF. You might want a practitioner who has the experience and ability to customize hormone replacement treatments. Since every patient is different, the practitioner should not have a set formula for dosing. While some natural hormones made by pharmaceutical companies are covered by insurance, these may only allow for modest tailoring. Compounded hormones can be tailored to you, but usually are not covered by insurance.

Additional Treatment Options

If you want additional treatment options, please order a copy of *Mold Warriors: Fighting America's Hidden Health Threat* by Shoemaker, Schaller and Schmidt from Amazon.com.

In the next chapter, you will see that even if you bathe in mold toxin binders, you will remain ill if you are continuously exposed to a moldy environment.

Treatment really must begin with removing water and mold from your home, school or workplace. Medical treatment that ignores solid and practical remediation is not in your best interest.

CHAPTER 13

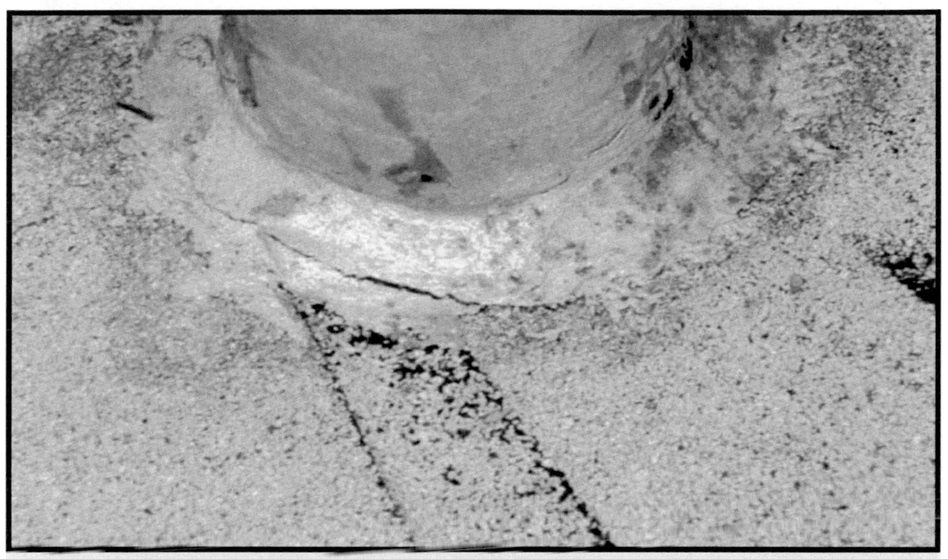

Here you can see cracks in the sealant around a pipe in the roof. This building had roof leaks and mold. Construction was never finished because the owner stopped paying for the defective work. There is a now a major lawsuit. Unless the builder goes out of business, the builder and/or his insurance company will have to pay for a third party to fix the mold problems and complete the building.

Smart and Ridiculous Mold Repairs and Clean-ups

We know that most mold remediations fail. And we know why. Because builders, mold remediation contractors, and insurance providers save money by taking shortcuts. Remediation work is rarely done right. Instead, problems are covered up and painted over.

Following water disasters, the insurance providers bring in their own network of out-of-state help (usually named "Bubba") to do the work. The insurance adjusters claim that these workers are all licensed. But what they don't tell you is that the license is a Fishing License!

Below we show five common cover-ups. What can you do about them? Make sure before any work is started that you see the license and the insurance policy of the contractor. Many states require special mold insurance for contractors doing mold work. General liability insurance *does not* cover mold-related work. Usually you can check out credentials of licensed contractors online with state contractor licensing. If they look fishy, bye-bye Bubba.

Wall Cavities

John's house has water damage from a burst pipe. John looks in the Yellow Pages and finds several local companies advertising mold work. He gets three quotes for the work, which he passes on to his insurance adjuster. All his quotes are around $8,000. But the insurance company has an affiliate company that can do the work for $4,000, since the insurance computer model says $4,000 is the fair, nationally-based pricing. The local pricing, the insurance company says, is out of line with national pricing because the local companies are all busy and charge too much.

Do you trust Bubba and the insurance company that sent him, or do you hire an attorney for a long costly fight?

John says, "Well, if the insurance company is recommending their affiliated mold contractor and says they are licensed and insured, they are probably fine."

John is literally "sick and tired" from the mold contamination in his home, so he just says, "Okay, come in and get started!"

John gives the go ahead. He did not check if Bubba or his company was licensed. He did not see if Bubba's company had at least $1 million in mold insurance coverage. He signs a little piece of paper to get things started, and in doing so, approves the choice of the company doing the work. The choice to use them is his—not the insurance company's.

Bubba does not remove any of the water-damaged walls. He claims that he is using a patented process where he sprays an enzyme on the wall surface that "is proven to penetrate into the wall cavities and kill all mold."

After Bubba leaves, John gets sick because the mold is still in the walls. He cannot sue the insurance company since he agreed to use Bubba. And the choice was his alone. And no, there is no real affiliation between Bubba and the insurance company. The insurance company claims they never recommended him. They claim their policy is to not make recommendations on remediation contractors.

Bubba is long gone ... back to Mississippi where he is cracking jokes: "Do you know how stupid those people in California are? Can you believe that they paid me $4,000 to spray 2 gallons of bleach on their walls? There is a sucker born every minute out there."

Cabinets

Most cabinet backs are made from pressed wood which is just glue and sawdust. Pressed wood works well unless it gets wet. When wet, this material absorbs moisture and is a preferred food source for many toxic molds. When the home is flooded from a break in a kitchen pipe, rarely will a company drying the house cut open or drill holes in the bottoms of the cabinets. However, this must be done in order to actively dry out this wet and enclosed space along with the wall cavity behind it.

If wet and not completely dried, the cabinet backs and bottoms along the wall behind need to be inspected to determine if there is a mold growth problem—usually this means cutting open a wall or cutting open cabinets.

Assume that most kitchen cabinets must be taken out and replaced if they got wet and were not quickly dried out.

We have never seen an insurance provider agree to this type of common sense care unless you exert a great deal of persistence. But persist you must. Also, consider shipping the ignorant insurance administrator your mold filled cabinets. After opening your loving gift, and after their hair falls out, perhaps they will be more reasonable with the next person.

Basements

Basements are part of your home. When they are moldy they usually contaminate the rest of the house.

Children should not play in moldy basements. Also, their toys and clothing should not be stored in the basement unless they are in sealed plastic bins.

In the real world, sometimes it is hard to make the basement mold-free. The next best thing is to:

☑ Minimize the mold in the basement;

☑ Minimize contamination of the rest of the home; and

☑ Keep children out of the problem area.

The home HVAC system should not be connected to a moldy basement. The problem basement should have its own HVAC system. The humidity in the basement should be kept under 65%. The HVAC system throughout the house should be equipped with MERV 11 HEPA filters to continuously clean the air of mold spores.

When Bubba comes out to your home, he will promise to rid your basement of mold (and remember, his promise is his word). But unless Bubba solves your moisture problem, the mold will always come back. It may not come back until the next rainy season when Bubba will be long gone, but it *will* come back. The only solution if there is continuous moisture is continuous removal of the mold spores by:

☑ Continuous air filtration. Put HEPA filters in your HVAC return grills and keep the HVAC fan turned to ON.

☑ Dilution with fresh air. The solution to pollution is dilution. Open your windows when you can.

☑ Venting the basement. The basement can often be vented to the outside.

☑ Using a portable dehumidifier to minimize the moisture and subsequent mold growth.

☑ Keeping the basement on its own separate HVAC system while constantly filtering the air with MERV 11 filters.

☑ Eliminating cardboard boxes, carpeting, curtains and fabric furniture in the basement area.

See our Appendix section on Problem Basements for more details.

HVAC and Ducts

Mrs. Homeowner is sick and calls an air duct cleaner to clean her ducts. Bubba the duct cleaner sprays an "EPA-approved" pesticide in the air duct. Sure, the pesticide he is using is approved ... to disinfect the floors of his hen house back home.

Know this: the EPA <u>does not</u> approve any pesticides for use in air ducts. Mr. Homeowner is now even sicker as a result of pesticide fumes.

If this occurs, consider calling a poison control center for immediate input. You also may want go to a respected emergency room, or be evaluated by a physician with a toxicology specialization, since different pesticides require highly diverse antidotes. If you go to your pediatrician or family physician, make sure your pesticide exposure is taken very seriously, since pesticides can be very dangerous immediately or over time.

Dr. Schaller often tests for pesticides and has found youth with both mold and pesticide exposure. Your local laboratory can send out 6 mls of blood to Specialty Labs, which can determine the type and level of pesticide or insecticide in you or your child. (The ordering details for your physicians include: Specialty Labs, pesticide/insecticide test, quantitative plasma screen, [3447], #S50444, and one possible diagnosis code is 293.9.)

Neurological signs and symptoms from pesticides in children are common. Some physicians believe activated charcoal capsules, sublingual glutathione, and NAC will help the liver remove low pesticide exposures. However, if pesticide is sprayed inside your home air ducts, it is best to find the exact name of the pesticide and the exact antidote.

Roof

Mr. Homeowner has mold in several areas of the home either from a roof leak or a leaking AC duct in the attic. He can't tell. His home is less than three years old. He calls out the builder's roofer who blames it on leaking AC ducts. Of course, the AC contractor says it is the roof.

The builder says, "We are sorry that your kids are all sick, you have lost your job, and your wife had to move in with her mother. We wish we could help, but the home warranty has expired and there is nothing we can do for you. Good luck."

Mr. Homeowner cannot afford a professional with an infrared thermographic camera to inspect his house in order to determine the source of the moisture problem. So he puts his house up for sale. In the meantime, he buys an air purifier for his sick daughter's room. He did not know that, as it kills some mold spores, the ozone produced by the purifier can permanently damage the lungs and cause migraines.

But this story has a happy ending. A friendly neighbor nicknamed "Fang" stopped by to ask about the *For Sale* sign. Fang is a top lawyer who sues builders for construction defects. Fang explained that there is a special extended warranty for building errors causing health problems called a "Statute of Repose" that typically covers the home up to 12 to 15 years. It covers construction defects that result in bodily harm. Clearly Mr. Homeowner and family are sick as a result of the construction defects.

Fang does not care if it is the fault of the AC contractor or the roofer because the builder is ultimately responsible. Let the builder sort out who is responsible.

Fang writes a short letter to the builder explaining that he has canvassed the neighborhood and found at least ten or twelve families with similar problems and was considering filing a class action suit. However, he explains to the builder that he is very, very busy suing fifteen other builders and would really prefer if the builder just took care of Mr. Homeowner who is his new best friend. The builder was given ten days to respond with his plan to cure the problem.

Low and behold the builder was at the house the next day, explaining that due to a lack of communication he was not really aware of their suffering, blah, blah, blah ... but in any event the home will be fixed by the end of the week.

Furthermore, a cleaning crew trained in mold remediation will come in and clean the home from top to bottom once the work is done. Legal help, more often than not, is required for builders to take your complaint seriously. If the builder is going to play dirty, sometimes you have to play dirty right back.

CHAPTER 14

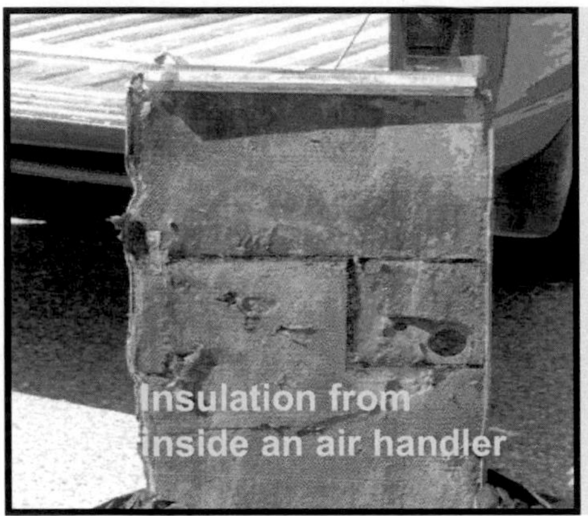

This insulation from the inside of an air handler is covered in black toxic mold (the original insulation color is light orange). Growth started due to a drain pan overflow and then spread like cancer. In this case, the mold in the air handler was not active during the summer because the AC was always on and, therefore, the air ducts were always too cold and dry for mold to thrive. But the mold went crazy in November when the residents first turned on the heat. Air sampling in the summer completely missed the problem.

The Dirty Little Secret that Heals: Air Conditioning Air Filters

Eddie is a very smart attorney. He defends doctors so he gets the best medical care in the state. He just had a shocking revelation about his mental fogginess and the moodiness of his children.

Eddie had no idea that simply taking care of his house can improve his health. He just discovered that the "air filters" inside his huge air conditioning & heating duct system have not been changed since he bought his home six years ago! He changes the air filters in his three ceiling return air grills about once a year, but only after they are so thick with dust that they are dark grey and make a whistling sound. But he did not know that there were also filters inside the actual indoor air handler units themselves, which was not the case in his last home.

When your Heating, Ventilation, and/or AC system (HVAC) has fresh, high quality air filters, it is like breathing a little slice of heaven. These filters have the ability to remove mold, contaminated dust, dust mites, animal dander, bacteria, viruses and other contaminants from your home. And they keep the HVAC duct system clean so mold cannot grow inside the system on duct dust. A fresh clean filter is truly your HVAC's best friend and essential for a healthy house.

We know we should change our toothbrush every month or two when the bristles are dingy. Likewise, we should replace our air filters just as frequently. Dirty air filters are a major blind spot in American health.

Clean Air Ducts

When you use high quality *disposable* air filters, your AC system and ducts stay clean.

When you throw them away, you discard the dirt, mold, and allergens that would normally be clogging up your lungs and your AC ducts. That is great for the homeowners, but horrible for air duct cleaners. They never get any business if high quality air filters are properly used, keeping the AC system clean.

AC people want to clean your ducts or sell you new air handlers when you destroy them by improper maintenance. They do not recommend quality disposable filters that you change yourself. Why? Because these decrease your need for air duct and AC cleaning! Did you think it was merely a coincidence that worthless, blue see-through filters are installed in your AC system when you purchase a home?

What Is The Right Filter?

Mike is a mold contractor. Weekly he hears from people who complain of "a few mold symptoms." They are not severely ill, but starting to be affected by a slightly elevated level of mold and related toxins. He had been telling such callers to replace every filter in their home with High Efficiency (HEPA) filters and to change them regularly. Amazingly, often that alone makes many feel better.

Mike has stopped making these recommendations since once people start using high quality filters, they rarely call him back for a mold remediation.

Be careful about using the blue junky filters and the complex permanent ones. Why? First, the blue junk filters are useless for controlling mold spores and do a very poor job at keeping your AC clean. Second, the "permanent" ones increase your exposure. You can expose yourself to billions of spores with one twist of the dirty filter on your way outside to clean it. As you carry it out of your home, you will be dispersing spores throughout your rooms like Johnny Appleseed throwing apple seeds.

The moral of the story? Use disposable filters. Put them immediately in sealed bags at the filter site while wearing a good "dust" mask that firmly covers your nose and mouth for the 10-20 seconds it takes to bag them. Have the bag open and ready so that the filter slips right into the bag as it comes out. A good mask is one that says "N-95" on the label. They are available at Home Depot or Wal-Mart for only a few dollars. You might feel this care is "over the top." But know this: there **almost always** will be a certain level of toxic chemicals in the filter dust. These chemicals have been used by at least two governments as biowarfare toxins. Why take the risk?

When you are shopping for an air filter, you should look for a "MERV" rating on the package. A MERV rating tells you the size of the holes that block the contaminants. The higher the MERV rating, the more filtration. And only the higher rated MERV filters do an excellent job cleaning the small particles, such as bacteria, allergenic dust mite feces, mold spores, and mold fragments from the air. Any reputable filter maker will have a MERV rating on the packaging. It might not jump out at you in five seconds, since some products have hundreds of words and scientific tables, but keep looking and you will find it.

MERV 11 filters do the best job at filtering out really small particles. These small particles are the ones that get trapped in the deepest and smallest air exchange sacks of the lungs.

On the next page is a chart that compares different types of air filters.

The type of filter we recommend is the 1" pleated electrostatic filter with a MERV 11 efficiency rating. These are available at Home Depot and some Wal-Mart stores.

filter comparison

We recommend using MERV 11

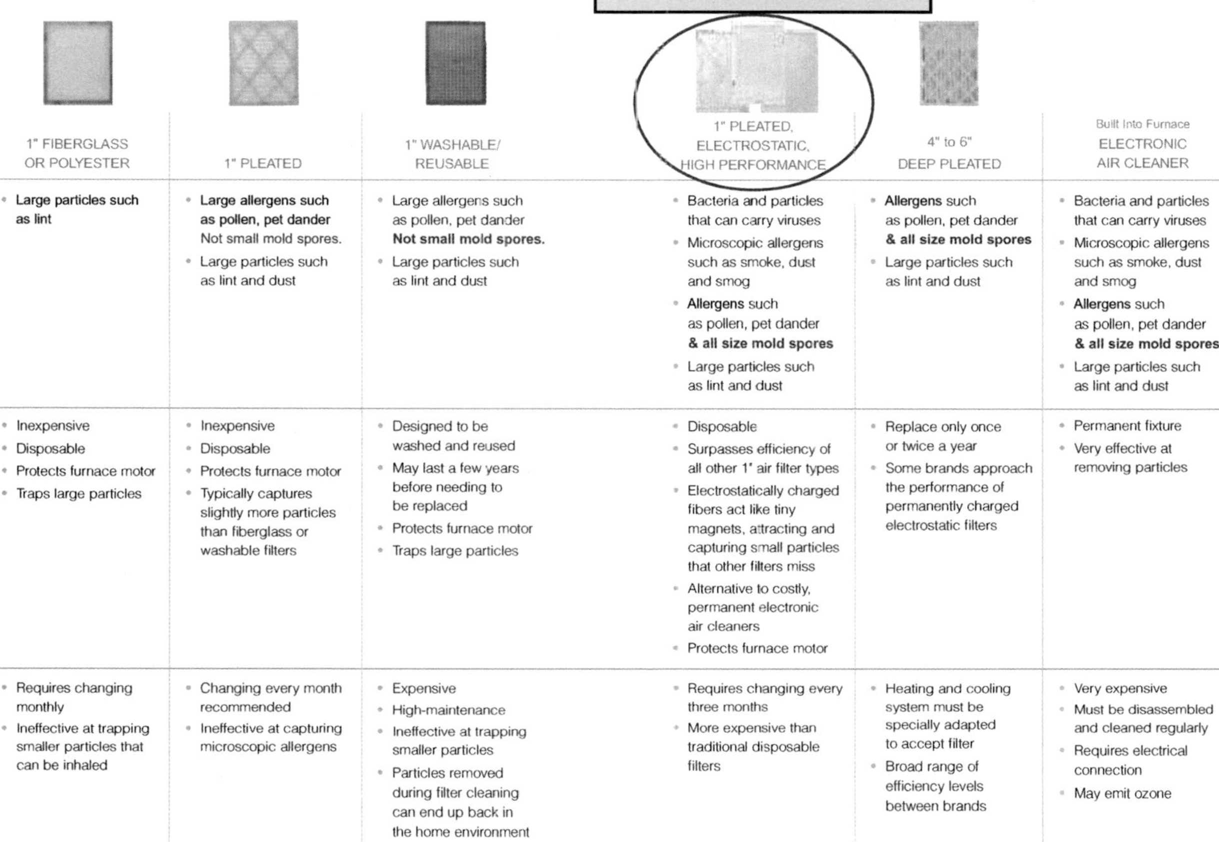

	1" FIBERGLASS OR POLYESTER	1" PLEATED	1" WASHABLE/ REUSABLE	1" PLEATED, ELECTROSTATIC, HIGH PERFORMANCE	4" to 6" DEEP PLEATED	Built Into Furnace ELECTRONIC AIR CLEANER
CAPTURES	• **Large particles such as lint**	• **Large allergens such as pollen, pet dander** Not small mold spores. • Large particles such as lint and dust	• Large allergens such as pollen, pet dander **Not small mold spores.** • Large particles such as lint and dust	• Bacteria and particles that can carry viruses • Microscopic allergens such as smoke, dust and smog • **Allergens** such as pollen, pet dander **& all size mold spores** • Large particles such as lint and dust	• **Allergens** such as pollen, pet dander **& all size mold spores** • Large particles such as lint and dust	• Bacteria and particles that can carry viruses • Microscopic allergens such as smoke, dust and smog • **Allergens** such as pollen, pet dander **& all size mold spores** • Large particles such as lint and dust
BENEFITS	• Inexpensive • Disposable • Protects furnace motor • Traps large particles	• Inexpensive • Disposable • Protects furnace motor • Typically captures slightly more particles than fiberglass or washable filters	• Designed to be washed and reused • May last a few years before needing to be replaced • Protects furnace motor • Traps large particles	• Disposable • Surpasses efficiency of all other 1" air filter types • Electrostatically charged fibers act like tiny magnets, attracting and capturing small particles that other filters miss • Alternative to costly, permanent electronic air cleaners • Protects furnace motor	• Replace only once or twice a year • Some brands approach the performance of permanently charged electrostatic filters	• Permanent fixture • Very effective at removing particles
CONSIDERATIONS	• Requires changing monthly • Ineffective at trapping smaller particles that can be inhaled	• Changing every month recommended • Ineffective at capturing microscopic allergens	• Expensive • High-maintenance • Ineffective at trapping smaller particles • Particles removed during filter cleaning can end up back in the home environment	• Requires changing every three months • More expensive than traditional disposable filters	• Heating and cooling system must be specially adapted to accept filter • Broad range of efficiency levels between brands	• Very expensive • Must be disassembled and cleaned regularly • Requires electrical connection • May emit ozone

When you have mold, bacteria, allergens, dander, or other contaminants in your home, and do not have MERV 11 class filters in your AC system, then your lungs filter these micro-particles from the air. Why would anyone suffering from allergies or any type of health problems want their lungs doing this instead of an air filter?

MERV 11: Use this quality if anyone in the home has allergies or if the home is old. Old homes inevitably have had leaks and water intrusions over the years. If the home clearly has mold, your new best friend is a MERV 11 air filter. So if you smell mold, see mold, or suspect your home has had water damage that was not fixed in two to three days, use a new MERV 11 air filter monthly.

MERV 8/9: Consider this lesser quality if you have no allergies or mold sensitivities and have a new and contaminant-free home. Such filters cost slightly less than the MERV 11s and allow the AC system to run a little more efficiently. They will also keep the AC clean.

A very convenient place to order any size filter is over the Internet at: *www.filters-now.com*. Filters can be ordered in custom sizes for a minimal extra charge.

How Often Do I Change Them?

It is time for healthy home care. If your home is dusty and moldy, you should change your air filters every 4 weeks. If your home is new and fairly clean, you can get by with changing them every 2 months.

If you see a layer of dust on the filter surface, do not wait until the mold spores hatch, grow through the filter, and start spreading through the house like cancer—toss it! Pitch it before it looks like a plant could grow on the surface.

And once you start using quality air filters, you will find that your house stays cleaner and requires less dusting.

Portable Air Purifies

In one large real estate facility, the ceiling tiles would get wet, moldy, and then be "replaced." When the maintenance guy popped out the old tiles, instead of discarding them, he would just leave them inside the ceiling so he did not have to carry the problem tiles through the office to discard. The ceiling over the office had, over time, 20-30 "discarded" moldy tiles just six to eight feet above the worker's desks.

> **Should I Use A Portable Air Cleaner?**
>
> **It has been proven in several recent studies that portable air cleaners actually do a very poor job of filtering the air in a room or office because they only effectively filter the air immediately around the air intake. They will only work well if the air in the room is well circulated. It is best to use a MERV 11 filter in the main AC. Your AC system was designed not only to cool/heat and filter the air, but also to provide efficient circulation through proper placement of supply and return air grills.**

Many of the office workers got sick. The building was tested for mold and found to be contaminated, but no one was sure how this could happen in a 2 year-old building. Each department purchased portable HEPA air cleaners for any employees complaining of mold-type illnesses. Once the air purifiers were installed (16 in all), most people claimed they felt somewhat better. But after a few weeks, everyone felt sick again. Why? The filters were completely clogged with dust. No one realized that these were not eternal filters. The cost to replace these custom filters was high (almost $75 per unit) and no one wanted to ask the boss to pay 16 x $75 for new air filters every month.

To make matters worse, two of the machines added to everyone's health problems. One continuously generated ozone, which can actually destroy lung tissue. The other problem machine was contaminated with mold and dispersed spores and mold toxins. What no one knew was that fitting the office's main AC system with a MERV 11 filter and turning the AC FAN to ON was equivalent to 65 portable machines!

When the AC FAN is ON, the air circulates throughout the office, filtering the air 24/7. When the FAN is OFF, the air is cleaned only when the AC system is running.

And replacing one large standard filter was about 65 times cheaper than buying the small custom filters needed for the portables.

A Simple & Helpful Intervention at Work or School?

One reason we wrote this book is to empower parents, teachers and employees to take back their health. We hope this short book will cause school and building owners to fix problems fast before people get ill and the school or property gets a bad reputation. School and building owners need to realize: "Fix water problems fast and save. Fight against the mold problems and lose."

Who handles the building filters? Your first action in dealing with a moldy school or building is to find the person in charge of filter maintenance. You and any others who are ill should befriend this person. Why? Their willingness to change the filters in the structure may control your health. Explain your experience and ask them to change the filtering. Mention that since some of the children, occupants and workers have severe allergies, you would appreciate having MERV 11 filters installed.

You may still need to pursue other appeals, including insurance, union and legal options in order to have the facility thoroughly remediated. But while you are fighting to get competent remediation—a process that is usually very slow and not always successful—keep the filters at high functioning to reduce the toxins your kids breathe.

Common Problems and Misconceptions Regarding "Air Conditioners"

Caroline is a trained engineer who was reading about air conditioning. She came across the term "air handlers" and was confused.

"I have no idea what an air handler does or where it is located. Everyone seems to assume this is common knowledge."

The air handler is the part of the air conditioning unit that cools the air and reduces indoor humidity as part of the cooling process. It is a large piece of metal equipment that is usually in the attic, basement, garage, or special closet. It sits in a wide part of the air duct system. Air ducts branch off from the air handler after the air is cooled. These ducts carry the cooled air all over your school or home. Return air ducts collect warmer air throughout the home, school or office, which is then sucked back to the air handler to start the air-cooling cycle again. (Some AC systems do not have return air ducts. Instead, the return air is sucked back into the AC system through a grill in either the door or the wall of the AC closet.)

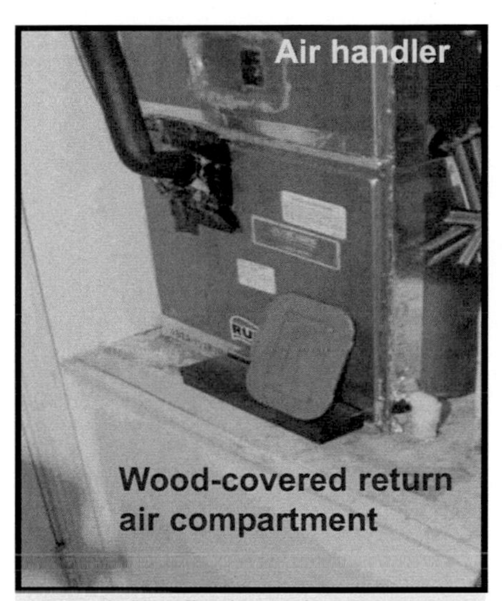

This air handler is not insulated well and water condensed on the metal surface, dripping down onto the wood return plenum below. In this case, the problem is only superficial and can be cleaned up by spraying the moldy wood with bleach.

The "condenser" is the part of the AC system that is always outside. It is where heat removed by the "air handler" is released.

Common AC Problems

Here are some common AC problems that may undermine the health of a school, home or business:

1. **Clogged drain**. When moist warmer air returns to the air handler and comes in contact with the cold air handler coils, water condenses on the coils. This water then drips onto the drain pan at the bottom of the air handler and then flows outside. This drainage pipe frequently becomes clogged with dust, algae, mold, and other debris. A flush with some bleach every season will not hurt the tubing and will prevent clogging. If you have your air handler serviced regularly by your AC company, make sure they clean the drain line.

The removal of a drainage pipe clog can be tricky and usually requires a $150 service call from your AC company. Better to use a little bleach each season in your line ... just like you use a little Drano in your sink to prevent it from clogging.

---

2. **AC is not controlling indoor humidity**. For some unknown reason, we are constantly coming across really dumb advice on the Web that people should set their AC thermostats to a high temperature, such as 82 degrees, to control indoor humidity. The opposite is true. If the AC does not run for extended periods of time, it does not reduce indoor humidity. When the AC is set to a low temperature such as 72 degrees, the AC coils will get cold enough so that moisture in the air condenses on the cooling coils. Water then drips off these coils and drains outside through the drain line, thereby drying the air. This is what dehumidifies indoor air.

3. **AC size too large?** There really is no such a thing as too large of an AC system. Here are the facts. The larger the AC capacity for a given building, the shorter the time the AC system runs to reach the temperature set on the thermostat. The shorter the run time, the less humidity the units are taking from the air as we mentioned above. A simple humidistat (Honeywell has one for $50-70 at Home Depot) connected to the AC thermostat will control the humidity in your home no matter how large the unit. The humidistat keeps the AC ON until the programmed humidity level (typically 65%) is reached.

   When your AC is controlled by a humidistat, it may occasionally get a bit chilly inside—especially on cooler humid days in the fall and spring—as your AC runs to keep the humidity at 65%. Wear a sweater.

   However, if your units are undersized and can't keep you cool in the summer or when you have a few extra people over, there is no simple fix. So keep your house cool for that July or August birthday bash with an AC unit that can easily cool your home when it is full of people on a hot summer day.

4. **Using cheap, see-through filters.** Good air filters keep the air handler and air ducts of your home free of dust. Dust grows mold, since it is a food source for mold. Mold does not grow on clean metal or clean AC ducts. Cheap filters do a poor job of keeping dust out of AC ducts.

5. **Don't keep the AC fan turned to ON?** We keep coming across more dumb advice that people should not keep their AC fan set to ON. When you have a MERV 11 HEPA filter in your AC system scrubbing your air, keep that fan on! The nonsensical argument about why you should keep your fan off is as follows: The AC coils in the air handler are wet. So if the AC fan runs while the AC is OFF and not cooling, then the fan will be blowing moisture off of the coils, adding humidity to the home.

   This could not be farther from the truth. First, if the humidity is under 65% mold will not grow. If the house humidity is set to 65% by the humidistat, then the AC fan is not increasing the indoor humidity because any moisture pushed into the house will be removed by the AC running a bit longer.

   Leaving the AC fan always ON increases air movement in the AC ducts, which actually reduces wet spots and mold growth inside the air ducts.

6. **Are ceiling fans worth installing?** After a shower, your bathroom humidity can be very high. Other rooms in your home can also become very warm or moist. Ceiling fans installed in all rooms of the house improve air movement, drying out moist closets and bathroom areas.

7. **Bathroom humidistat controlled exhaust fans**. A Honeywell $50-70 humidistat connected to your bathroom exhaust fan can be set to automatically run your exhaust fan when the humidity exceeds 65%, like after a hot shower.

8. **Drain pan overflow alarm**. Most new homes have a sensor connected to the air handler drain pan that is located below the air handler. If the drain clogs, the sensor sets off an alarm so you

can fix the problem *before* you have water overflowing the drain pan and causing a mold disaster. If you do not have such an alarm, we recommend having one installed.

CHAPTER 15

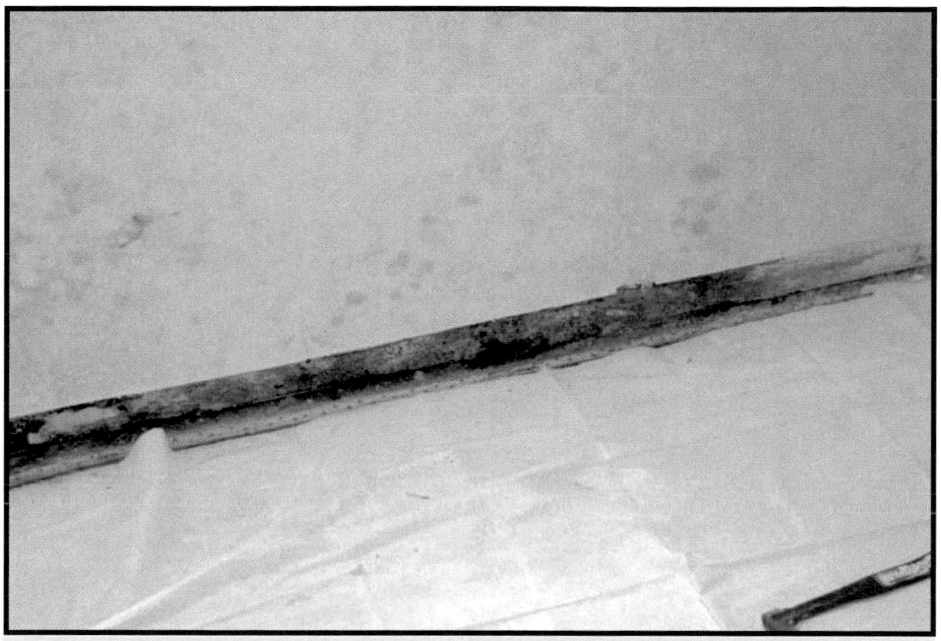

After removing the baseboard, we found hidden black mold on the wall behind. In all cases, if the baseboard has any water staining, it should be removed to see if there is any indication that there could be toxic mold growing in the wall behind.

Professional Mold Investigation and Remediation

Before hiring someone to test or remediate your home or office, you should know some basics on mold testing, cleaning and remediation. If you ask a tester or remediator about EPA or OSHA guidelines and they have never heard of them, hire a different remediator.

Does a Professional Mold Remediation Plan Make Sense?

If you have access to a computer, you can read basic mold remediation and clean up principles at: *www.epa.gov/mold.* After you read this material, you should be able to tell if a mold remediation plan makes sense.

Size Matters

If you have a small mold source, it can be repaired with less drama than if your home was flooded for a week. But some principles will always apply even to the smallest mold remediation. For example:

1. No moldy object should ever be carried through your home or school unless it is fully sealed in plastic wrap or a plastic garbage bag. Ideally, it should be pushed out an open window (if you are on the ground floor).
2. The smallest movement or vibration of a moldy surface during cleaning can result in literally billions of toxin-filled spores being released into the air. Before removing moldy materials, the area should be sealed with plastic curtains, and there should be a fan in the window pointed out and turned on to HIGH.
3. Remediators who are not wearing any face, mouth, hand, or body protection in the midst of visible mold or moldy odors are untrained and should be asked to leave. You will be hurt by their lack of training.
4. The focus of repairs should include finding the exact source(s) of the water that caused the damage. We often see reports of mold remediators that show no awareness or focus on fixing the source of the water. If your home is 100% cleaned of all mold, but leak(s) continue, the mold will always return. The remediator should have an understanding of building defects that lead to water leaks or condensation. The plan should start with removing all water problem sources, which are always the cause of mold growth. An infrared thermographic camera is a device that can help locate excess humidity and water behind walls and ceilings. It is expensive and most mold assessors or mold remediators will not have one.
5. Before removing moldy materials, remediators should seal, trap or capture as much surface mold growth as possible to prevent the spread of toxic spores. How?

a. They can carefully damp clean moldy surfaces with a disinfectant. This will remove and capture as much surface growth as possible before it can fly into the air. Mold spores and dust can be captured by HEPA vacuuming and damp cleaning, but never by sweeping, dry dusting or brushing.

b. Hard-surfaced porous materials, such as concrete or cement walls and floors, should be disinfected with bleach diluted one part bleach to ten parts water or stronger. However, this should be done only after cleaning away any visible mold or dirt; otherwise, the bleach will be useless in killing deeper mold. The solution should be applied by light misting or wiping on to avoid runoff. The entire area that supported visible growth, as well as the surrounding area, should be fully treated. The surfaces should be kept damp with the solution for at least 30 minutes (ideally up to two hours), rinsed and then allowed to air dry. Since diluted bleach is a very poor cleaning agent, and is inactivated by organic matter, it is critical to thoroughly clean off major visible growth and soiling before bleaching with diluted bleach. (Straight bleach, rather than diluted bleach, can do a very good job of removing built-up mold on concrete, wood trusses, or siding, but special equipment is required to protect workers from the strong fumes.)

c. Porous materials, such as dry wall or carpet, should be enclosed in tight plastic sheeting or bags and discarded if they have visible mold growth or strong mold odors.

d. Non-porous materials, such as solid wood, metal, plastic, concrete, or tile, should be thoroughly cleaned of all visible mold growth and dirt by scrubbing with an all-purpose cleaner or detergent solution. For final wiping, use clean water with a disinfectant in it. Straight bleach (Clorox) will destroy mold, mold spores and mycotoxins, and is a very good mold cleaner when it can be used safely on a material.

e. Fabrics items, such as clothes, furniture, curtains, etc., can be saved if washed fully and carefully. Clothes should be washed in a washing machine with detergent or dry cleaned if they are not machine-washable. However, machine washing is preferable. Add bleach to the wash if it will not damage the clothes. Unless there is actual mold growth on a fabric item, such as a sofa, fabric can always be cleaned by some combination of washing with detergent, HEPA vacuuming, dry cleaning, and/or on-site steam cleaning.

f. Through human foot traffic and AC ducts, a moldy area can contaminate nearby and distant rooms. Cleaning must take into account that mold spores and contaminated dust can be widely and easily dispersed. The problem remediated area, as well as all other contaminated areas, should be carefully cleaned. For example, if a bathroom wall had mold, it should be assumed that the carpet leading out of the bathroom has extensive mold spores and mold toxins in the dust. Similarly, the ducts removing air from the problem bathroom will move contaminated air to all areas serviced by that air handler. All these areas need special cleaning.

6. All remediated materials must be completely dried of all moisture from cleaning activities or disinfectant solutions. Dehumidifiers, fans, and ventilation with dry warm air are used to speed drying.

7. If the water damage was caused by unclean water such as a flood or toilet overflow, call in professionals. Do not attempt to do the work yourself. The EPA guidelines are only meant for small problems involving clean water. For large or significant problems, call in a professional.

Our sister publication, *Mold Remediation: What You Must Know Before You Hire a Remediation Contractor* provides complete information on effective mold remediation.

Guidelines for Professional Mold Investigation

Mold inspectors like to take many, many measurements and samples. The more measurements and samples they take, the more scientific they appear. But most of these are rarely of any practical value for mold remediation.

Mold growth is the problem indicator we care about. If mold is growing, then excess moisture and food sources are available. Mold is nature's indicator of a moisture problem. Indoor mold growth is always a sign of a mold problem, regardless of the species of mold.

Useful Terminology

Air-O-Cell Cassettes: Provides a snap shot of the total amount of mold spores in the air. This air sampling methodology does not tell you the species of mold, only the basic types (genus) of mold found. Rarely does a homeowner need to know the species of mold.

Anderson/Bio Cassettes: Collects air samples and then allows you to culture and determine the actual species of mold, such as *Aspergillus fumigatus*. *Fumigatus* is the species; *Aspergillus* is the genus. Some feel this may help legally and medically. But for legal and medical cases, we strongly suggest DNA analysis (called Quantitative PCR analysis).

Swabs/tape: Allows one to determine the kind of mold growing on a surface. This is rarely useful as professionals usually can tell visually if something that looks like mold growth is, in fact, mold. And, generally, we do not care which type of mold is growing because, according to the EPA, all indoor mold growth should be eliminated. The exception is determining if dust in AC ducts or plenums is contaminated with mold. This is often hard to determine visually without lab confirmation.

Equipment

An infrared thermographic camera can be very useful to trace the source of moisture causing mold growth. Laser particle counters can determine immediately the locations of elevated particle levels so you can trace the source of contamination. Both of these tools are excellent. And both are often required for a competent evaluation and remediation plan.

Most mold inspectors do not have an infrared thermographic camera or a laser particle counter. They try to make up for this by taking every other kind of reading imaginable: air sampling, CO2, CO, moisture, humidity, temperature, etc. Then they write big reports explaining why the data collected means such and such, and why they can't find the source of the problem or verify that any problems even exist. And by the way, here's the invoice. Please pay promptly.

☑ **Visible mold or mold smells are certain and clear indicators that there is a problem with a building.** Testing of any kind should only be done if it helps determine the extent of the mold problem and how to fix it. If someone suggests testing of any kind, it is important to ask why. In almost all cases, consultants use readings and results from moisture meters, air sampling, tape lifts, mold swabs, CO2, CO, etc., to cover up the fact that they have no idea how to go about fixing the mold problem.

☑ If there is no visible mold but hidden mold is suspected because of mold odors or sick occupants, air sampling can be very useful. Due to cost concerns, usually a mold inspector will only take 2-3 samples, even for a 4,000-sq ft. house. However, many air samples (5-10) often will need to be taken in different parts of the home or office to find elevated mold levels associated with hidden mold. For example, if an office or bedroom has 10 times the *Aspergillus/Penicillium* mold spore count as the rest of the house, you can deduce that the water source is or was most likely nearby. At this point, having an infrared camera, a laser particle counter, and building experience are useful for finding the exact location of the water source and mold.

☑ Moldy smells mean hidden mold. As you know, sometimes you can smell the mold and at other times that mold smell is just not there. For the same reason, when you test for mold, sometimes it is there to be found by testing and sometimes it is not. Air sampling can give false negatives. But find the water source and either you will find the mold or there will be mold growing shortly.

☑ **Sick people with mold toxin symptoms or abnormal blood labs are often the best indicators of mold growth. The human body's sensitivity routinely beats mold testing.** Testing is a snapshot of the air at a particular time, but sickness is from a long-term accumulation of problems. Because of this, mold-related symptoms and medical lab reports are often more reliable than mold air sampling.

Remember that the typical training for a mold tester/investigator is 2-3 days of classroom training, none of which is actually on-site mold testing in real situations.

The American Industrial Hygiene Association (AIHA) recommends that, at a minimum, individuals conducting mold investigations should possess a bachelor's degree in a relevant science: industrial hygiene, biology, chemistry, chemical, environmental or mechanical engineering, physics, environmental health, or safety. They should also have advanced training in:

- Indoor Environmental Quality;
- Microbiological Assessment and Remediation based on current standards, such as those published by IESO (*www.IEStandards.org*);
- Heating, Ventilation, and Air Conditioning (HVAC); and
- Building Science.

This background is rarely found in mold investigators and, therefore, they are not able to get mold insurance coverage. Mold investigators without the adequate background, training, and mold insurance are rarely effective.

Qualified individuals will have mold insurance; non-qualified individuals will not. As a result, checking for mold insurance can be very useful. If they do not have any mold insurance, their lack of qualifications will be your disaster.

If you cannot find someone who knows what they are doing for the price you can afford, consider doing the testing yourself. There are several companies (including our own) that will loan out professional air sampling equipment (by UPS) and walk you through the testing. Email Dr. Rosen at hometest@mold-free.org for more information on his tester loaner program.

Our sister publication, *Locating Hidden Toxic Mold: What You Need to Know Before Hiring a Mold Investigator or Buying Real Estate*, provides complete education on how to locate mold in your home or office.

CHAPTER 16

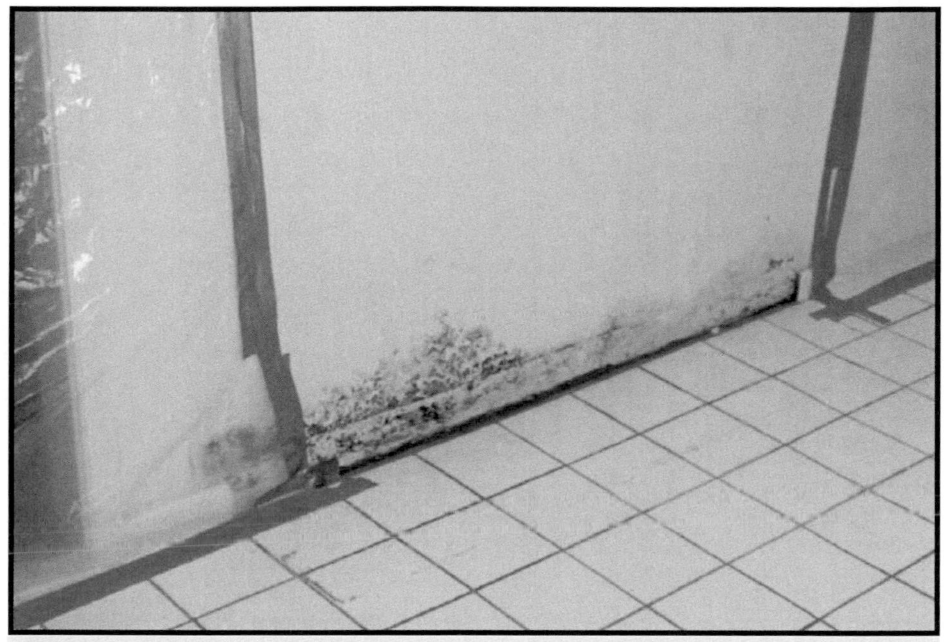

We found *Stachybotrys*, a highly toxic "black mold," behind built-in cabinets. In general, when you find some *Stachybotrys* on a wall surface, you will find even more inside the wall, since *Stachy* grows relatively slowly and needs ample moisture present for an extended period of time.

Laboratory Testing for Biotoxin Symptoms: Beyond Simple Allergy Labs

Many physicians and patients think that mold merely affects your nasal areas and lungs. So they think a "full laboratory" evaluation is simply allergy testing and perhaps some special breathing tests called "Pulmonary Function Tests." While these have a use, they are limited tests and miss the point that mold toxins are

always active throughout the **entire** human body, possibly affecting all organs or systems.

Below we review select and special lab tests that are used to check for mold toxin symptoms. Your family doctor could order these tests if you are concerned about mold exposure. Although very important, these tests are not commonly done. They should be.

We are not trying to turn you into "little doctors," and so we will try to avoid medical jargon. But some of these lab tests and explanations can be a little technical. What matters most is that you get the test. After that, you can explore any abnormal result with your physician.

Children usually prefer getting as little blood work as possible. The use of a compounded pain relieving cream or prescription EMLA cream can reduce pain if applied an hour before blood testing. We also routinely use 0.5 mg of Xanax to calm frightened children. They are very thankful.

In a perfect world, we would suggest large adolescents and adults get as many of the lab tests as possible. Below we discuss several of the most important ones for children.

What is important about blood testing? Blood tests can be used to both diagnose biotoxin exposure and follow the success of treatment for exposure. However, without removing the person from the toxic environment, medical treatments will not be fully successful.

Melanocyte Stimulating Hormone (MSH)

Perhaps one of the most serious blind spots in current medical practice is an ignorance of the massive role that MSH plays in the body. It is a major controlling hormone involved in up to twenty functions. If it is low, a child, teacher or parent could have any one of thirty different problems. It is not an optional lab test, and I (Schaller) feel it should be part of an average medical work-up in all Americans. The most common cause of a very low MSH in my patients is exposure to biotoxins. If it is below 35 according to LabCorp ranges, it is low. And many youth with biotoxin exposure can have less than 20. In addition to mold toxins, Lyme or Babesia biotoxins and severe inflammation also can reduce MSH levels.

You might recall from high school biology that MSH is involved in skin color. Now we know it has many other serious health roles in the body. In fact, pharmaceutical companies around the world are seeing the many roles for this hormone and are scrambling to make it in a slightly altered form so they can patent it. They expect to make a fortune.

So what do all these drug companies know? What role does MSH have besides tanning and skin color?

MSH's Expanded Roles

MSH has many roles, but a low MSH does not mean a child will have all the problems listed below.

Memory and learning: If your child has a low MSH, then they will have a harder time recalling class work. A child with a low MSH may seem forgetful and may struggle to stay on top of school work.

I wonder, how many children across America receive special education because of a reduced MSH? Since this is not normative medicine, we do not know yet. But it appears quite common in our patients with mold toxin poisoning or tick-borne Lyme disease.

Mold Toxin Poisoning & ADD/ADHD

While true ADD or ADHD exists, most child experts are not aware of the role that biotoxins from sick buildings plays in creating behaviors that resemble these disorders. Some young children lose these problems when they move out of their sick home or school. In these cases, we would say they had "secondary" ADD or ADHD. The parent, teacher or pediatrician was not hallucinating. There was more to the child's behavior than "ants in the pants" or just "being a boy." But the behavior problem was from mold toxins—not from genetics, an intrauterine exposure, or injury as in primary ADD or ADHD.

Attention will fall in children or adults as MSH drops. I have repeatedly had patients called "ADHD" or "ADD," but these symptoms often started after they were fourteen years old. ADHD and ADD do not suddenly start in adolescence!

Obesity (or too thin): Typically, children and adults with a low MSH gain weight. Often they gain a significant amount of weight. Perhaps some people try to feel better by eating. But others gain weight with only moderate eating. Commonly, people with low MSH see their weight drift higher and higher. Diets may help somewhat, but people do not get the results they expect from their diet. They lose five pounds instead of fifteen. A small number of people struggle to maintain their body fat and start to look waif-like. (It may be that they exercise massive amounts to create natural opioids to feel better.)

Pain relief: MSH encourages production of your natural opioids. If your MSH is low, you will feel aches and pains more often. Some youth complain of headaches. Others report joint pain, which is often called "growth pains." Further, you may be more inclined to do addictive, impulsive or pleasurable behaviors, in an effort to feel "normal" or "right" again. These addictive behaviors are very diverse. Low MSH promotes alcoholism, illegal drug use, binge eating, sexual experimentation, impulsive exercise, intense work, speed driving, thrill-seeking actions, pornography addiction, and rage. With binge work, a person does not want to stop working because once they stop, they do not feel "right." Impulsive activity also may create a small amount of natural pain-killing chemicals. And patients with rage may feel briefly "better" after a "blow-up" for a similar reason.

Flat or bored mood: Having an MSH deficiency can reduce your feeling of joy. A person can be left with a malaise that is often different than typical depression.

Increased inflammation: MSH has strong affects on inflammation chemicals. If MSH drops, it will allow inflammation chemicals to increase. Inflammation causes increased pain, a depressed or irritable mood, increased agitation and increased blood clots that may increase heart attacks and strokes. Low MSH also is associated with an increase in lung inflammation or asthma, in addition to inflamed intestinal disorders.

Decreased coping ability: Low MSH makes it hard for body organs and the brain to handle stresses, e.g., personal stresses or toxin exposures.

Energy changes: In our experience, some patients with low MSH have increased fatigue and are listless. Some patients have both agitation and fatigue simultaneously.

Nerve repair: Throughout his or her life, the average person suffers many injuries that can hurt neurons—falls, car accidents, sports accidents, and simple aging. In addition to these, it appears low MSH may slow nerve repair.

Low libido or erection problems: Both genders have a significant drop in free testosterone in their 40s. For some it is over a 50% drop. This can make sex as interesting as a sewer. Men with a low MSH can also find that their plumbing is not functioning, not merely because of low testosterone or very low estrogen, which can cause a low libido, but because they have abnormally low MSH. For libido, women need a little testosterone, estrogen and progesterone. But if MSH is low, these hormones usually are also impaired, and libido can be affected. While a low libido might be good for adolescents, it is not a "benefit" one can pick with a low MSH—you get other negatives.

Excessive urination or mouth dryness: While this is often seen as a sign of diabetes, few physicians realize a low MSH can also cause this annoying symptom. Children dislike having to go more than their friends and looking peculiar. Also, this unique form of urination removes salt from the body. Others have uncomfortable dry mouths that do not respond well to treatment.

Body temperature: Some children or adults have flashes of hot or cold sensations.

Testing MSH

Please do not go to just any laboratory. LabCorp offers the most meaningful clinical results. If you want a doctor to order a test for you, you will need to have all the material in this chapter in hand. And you will particularly need the material below, which lists the test codes and the name of the special kits needed. LabCorp patient locations for a useful MSH can be found on the Internet at: *www.LabCorp.com.*

Please make sure the lab has a special test kit in stock before you go—the Trasylol kit.

Most physicians would not have the training to do this test in their office. So if an office clerk says they can, I would ask if they have any "Trasylol kits" in stock to be sent to LabCorp. After this blows them away, perhaps they might realize they are not equipped and will send you to a local LabCorp center.

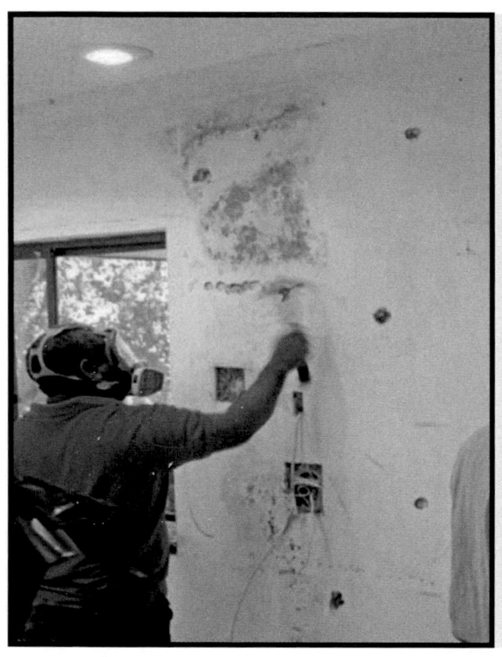

An ill housewife smelled mold in the kitchen. The husband thought she was "nuts." After extensive testing, it was confirmed that there was a hidden mold problem in the kitchen walls. To understand and eventually fix the problem, the kitchen cabinets, including the marble countertop, had to be removed. The walls behind the cabinets were covered with mold. Insurance only paid a fraction of the cost to repair. But the wife returned back to work 3 weeks later after being on disability for 4 years!

Does MSH Replacement Exist?

Currently, the use of bio-identical MSH is not FDA-approved. While a form exists that is a human, rat and mouse form—it is the same in all three mammals—it is not available for clinical use. Amazingly, the National Institutes of Health are not making MSH research a priority. Yet, many drug companies are scrambling to get patents. China is making this in many different factories. And an Australian pharmaceutical company has invented a patch delivery form. Hopefully, some drug company will have this approved in the USA soon, and patients with MSH deficiency will be able to use a patch or transdermal cream to replace their low MSH. Of course, many patients have their MSH return to normal after using Cholestyramine toxin-binding agent and staying out of moldy homes or schools.

HLA DRB, DBQ Disease Evaluation Made Simple

Do not be overwhelmed by this confusing name. Let us make it simple. As you know, if you need a transplant, like a kidney, it is better to get it from a relative who has similar cell surface proteins.

After doctors were matching organ transplants for a while, scientists noticed that some cell surface proteins seemed to be found in certain diseases. So these cell markers or cell "clothing" were expanded to disease testing. If a person had a certain pattern, they were at higher risk to develop a certain disease. Using our clothing analogy, a person wearing black leather is rarely a kindergarten teacher. The clothes "make" or give us insight into the man, and the cell's outer markers or "clothing" give us insight into the cell.

Dr. Shoemaker used this testing in thousands of patients and found very clear patterns regarding mold toxin removal. He found that about twenty-five percent of the U.S. population does not properly remove mold toxins. So if they are exposed to even just low levels of mold toxins, toxins are collected in their bodies and over time can make these individuals more and more ill.

We found the same patterns and they fit exactly with a child's medical troubles. This is very progressive medicine, and slowly more and more physicians are learning how to do this type of analysis.

We are very pleased to offer a reading of your HLA results, which will be done by both Dr. Schaller and Dr. Shoemaker. So for $35.00, you will have two prolific, creative research physicians read your HLA pattern, and send back a chart with your pattern circled clearly. The money will be used to fund further health care publications by the Shoemaker and Schaller team.

In the book *Mold Warriors: Fighting American's Hidden Health Threat*, there are some tools for interpreting the HLA patterns. But some folks want clear coaching in reading their results.

Simply send your results to Dr. Schaller.

Fax Number: 239-304-1987

Mailing Address: Professional Medical Services of Naples
Community Bank Towers
Suite 305
5150 Tamiami Trail North
Naples, Florida 34103

Enclose a check for $35 made out to: James Schaller, M.D.

Or go to the *www.personalconsult.com* home page and pay $35.00 by credit card where it reads, "Make a payment." Allow fourteen days for processing, since either doctor may be away at conferences.

Dr. Schaller will read it first and forward it to Dr. Shoemaker for a second opinion. In the rare event only one physician is able to read your test, due to illness or international travel, we feel you will still get a solid result.

The test name and LabCorp code is: HLA DRB, DBQ Disease Evaluation 012542. Some physicians use these diagnostic codes: 279.10, 377.34, 279.8.

Leptin

Leptin is made by fat cells and is supposed to stop fat production and reduce appetite. Many things can interfere with proper Leptin function. For example, leptin function is often affected by biotoxins. Mold biotoxins ultimately cause leptin resistance, meaning that leptin does not work on its receptor. As a result, the body makes much more than it needs and your blood levels shoot up. So leptin levels commonly become abnormal in a person who cannot remove mold toxins. These individuals become bloated and puffy and have trouble losing weight. They might lose some weight with great effort, but not as much as they should.

Sick Building Syndrome often causes blood leptin to go far above the normal range. If you or your child is no longer exposed to mold toxins, the leptin level should go down on its own. Taking Cholestyramine at one to two doses/day for children and four doses/day for adults for an appropriate period after the mold exposure is gone can also lower leptin levels. Furthermore, you can measure leptin levels to track your improvement—it should fall as you remove mold toxins from your body and avoid moldy schools and homes. If it does not return to normal, consider a consultation with a physician who specializes in mold toxin removal. You can get this test at any lab and one possible diagnostic code is 253.2.

Myelin Basic Protein

Myelin is the fat insulation on nerves. Mold and Lyme toxins can cause this insulation to be attacked by your own antibodies.

Sometimes this is misdiagnosed as M.S.

The immune system loses control and makes antibodies that hurt the fatty nerve protection. This lab must be done at Specialty Labs and is easily sent out from LabCorp and Quest labs. The Specialty Lab code is 848747 with a possible diagnostic code of 340.

We have seen good results in restoring fatty nerve protection after mold remediation and mold medical care. And others improved still further with the treatment of commonly missed infections, such as Lyme, Bartonella, Ehrlichia, Babesia and Mycoplasma. Lyme, for example, can be hidden inside a wide range on human cells, which probably increases autoimmunity.

Anticardiolipin (IgA, IgG & IgM)

This lab test measures antibodies against a very specific type of cell wall fat called phospholipids. An abnormal lab result means you are attacking your own cell walls, which can cause deadly blood blots, strokes and heart attacks, and abortions.

Antigliadin Antibodies

Gliadin is a wheat protein that can cause intestinal irritation in some susceptible people. If mold toxins get into the body, the inflammation system can rise, causing a possible sensitivity to wheat and other common grains. Generally, after indoor mold exposure, the lab results might show the beginning of antibodies against gliadin, but the patient may not have diarrhea or severe intestinal problems yet. Any lab can do this test.

ANA with Reflex

This tests if the mold toxins have caused you to start making antibodies against your own cell nuclear material. If positive, the "reflex" means they run other tests to find out the specific types of anti-antibodies that are present. This can be done by any lab and is known to most progressive physicians.

Homocysteine

Mold toxins sometimes consume B-Vitamins, which causes a rise in homocysteine. Most sincere physicians do not realize indoor mold can increase this dangerous amino acid. A high homocysteine triggers inflammation, injury to blood vessels, and dangerous blood clotting. This lab test is well known to physicians.

IgE

If a child or adult has asthma or allergies to a mold, the IgE level will be high. But in general, mold toxins have very little effect on IgE. If it is high, an allergist, pulmonologist, ENT, pediatrician, or family doctor could probably offer some relief, since this is a common and well-known medical problem. The toxins of mold do not cause it.

Epstein Barr Panel

We all have been exposed to this virus. So, it is assumed everyone will have results showing its presence in the blood. Some physicians feel a very high number means your immune system is not acting normally due to mold toxins or some infection hurting the immune system. Any lab can do this test. The LabCorp code is 010280 and a possible diagnostic code is 780.79.

Lab Tests Done By Quest Labs

If possible, these next two lab samples would need to be packaged in dry ice and shipped overnight to: Quest Diagnostics, 1901 Sulphur Spring Rd., Baltimore, Maryland 21227. Their phone number is 410-536-1324. Some LabCorp centers or local Quest centers will agree to send these out to Quest.

VEGF

This hormone helps make new capillaries and increases blood, oxygen and sugar flow to various tissues, including the brain and muscle tissue. Some mold toxins cause abnormal levels of VEGF—either low levels or huge levels much higher than the maximum of the normal range. Either extreme is bad. Three common symptoms of abnormal VEGF are atypical muscle aches after exertion, fatigue and brain fog. All are likely due to the inability of VEGF to open capillaries to deliver oxygen and perhaps also glucose to the body. Abnormal levels are partially treated with high doses of Omega-3 fish oils. The Quest code is 894826 and some possible diagnosis codes are 416.9, 253.2, 710.0.

Also, any youth with excessive fatigue should be tested for an infection which is commonly missed—Babesia. It is typically passed on to people through very tiny ticks, which inject pain killers and antihistamines along with the Babesia infection. Therefore, a youth with significant fatigue should have an IGeneX Babesia FISH test done along with an IgG and IgM. Some physicians think that Babesia will commonly produce urine tests showing burst red blood cells. Unfortunately, this is not always true in mild American forms. Sometimes a child can have no signs or symptoms for years.

MMP-9

This enzyme goes up with the presence of tumors, sudden severe infections, significant inflammation and biotoxin release. Exposure to toxic mold chemicals will increase the MMP-9 level, typically over 300.

It should decrease as the child or adult improves from treatment for toxin exposure. The Quest code is 821675, and one possible code is 340.

Mold with Lyme Disease

The number one vector illness in the U.S. is Lyme disease. It is found in every state, but one study showed that only 1 in 40 positive cases is reported to state agencies. The disease is carried by ticks that are often no bigger than a poppy seed and are rarely visible (unlike the large ticks found on dogs).

We have found that some patients have *both* mold toxin illness and Lyme disease. Typically, this condition is missed because of the use of improper or inadequate laboratory testing.

If you want to rule out Lyme, consider using IGeneX labs, which is a Medicare CLIA-approved lab with exceptional blind negative and blind positive results. They do not use a single Lyme test strain from Europe or a single state. They also do not exclude key search proteins because of legal patents. Rather, they grow out and harvest the Lyme so that they offer equal and complete amounts of Lyme's proteins. The tests use these proteins to bind to your antibodies. Furthermore, IGeneX's blind testing is far better than the published results of many labs. So, if you are relying on a lab which doesn't use proteins specific for Lyme strains found throughout the USA, good luck!

We have seen individuals who had vivid bull's-eye rashes from Northern states come back fully negative after 1-5 months. They had clear symptoms that were not treated and were positive with IGeneX testing. Why mention this material? Some people have been exposed to mold and pick up a tiny poppy-seed-sized deer tick along the way. So, they have mold illness and Lyme. You can order a test kit and mailer from IGeneX at 800-832-3200.

Dr. Schaller is writing a pediatric tick-borne infection book with a Connecticut pediatrician who has treated 9,000 children with Lyme and other tick infections. In the meantime, for more information, log onto Dr. Schaller's web site, *www.personalconsult.com*, for over 140 Lyme disease articles.

Other Labs For Future Blood Draws

We realize that many children, as well as adults, do not like undergoing a large number of blood tests. However, if the patient is willing and physically able to take them, the following lab tests can be useful in diagnosing mold-related health problems.

Complement 3a or C3a

This chemical is increased during pregnancy, perhaps to increase a mother's ability to fight infection. It is a strong pro-inflammation chemical acting in at least two inflammation systems. It is seen increased in everything from unstable heart chest pain to aspirin-induced asthma. Have the samples sent to Quest Labs in Baltimore or any lab that can perform the test. The lab code is C3 4859W with a possible diagnosis of 279.8.

Vasoactive Intestinal Polypeptide (VIP)

This chemical is a very strong agent in dampening immune reactivity. Some research shows that it even stops multiple-sclerosis-like damage and reduces cell death by decreasing granzyme, perforin and FasL. It may soon have a role in treating patients with autoimmunity, excess immune reactivity, and organ transplants. The test can be performed by LabCorp and requires the special chilled trasylol tube used in MSH tests. The lab code is 010397 with possible diagnostic codes of 787.91, 259.9 and 780.8.

Future Blood Lab Research

In the previous chapters, we discuss numerous tests that might be beneficial for adult diagnosis, but are rarely prescribed for children. Sample additional lab tests for adults include interleukins, inflammatory cytokines, cardiac C-reactive protein, and apolipoproteins. In the near future, we hope to evaluate more closely a dozen autoimmune tests, a dozen special hormones, the kinin system, acetylated peptide A, PAR-2 (and related products), granzyme, perforin, and hemolysin in very select patients who are not improving.

Endnotes

[1]Storey, E., Dangman, K. H., DeBernardo, R. L., Yang, C. S., Bracker, A., Hodgson, M. J. 2004. *Guidance for Clinicians on the Recognition and Management of Health Effects Related to Mold Exposure and Moisture Indoors*. University of Connecticut Health Center. September, 2004.

[2]*Lett Appl Microbiol*. 2005;41(4):367-73; Comparison of populations of mould species in homes in the UK and USA using mould-specific quantitative PCR; US Environmental Protection Agency, Cincinnati, OH 45268, USA. vesper.stephen@epa.gov

[3]*Adv Appl Microbiol*. 2004;55:191-213; Possible role of fungal hemolysins in sick building syndrome; Vesper SJ, Vesper MJ; U.S. Environmental Protection Agency Office of Research and Development, National Exposure Research Laboratory 26 W. M. L. King Drive Cincinnati, Ohio 45268, USA.

[4]*Environ Monit*. 2004 Jul;6(7):615-20. Epub 2004 May 26; Quantitative PCR analysis of house dust can reveal abnormal mold conditions; Meklin T, Haugland RA, Reponen T, Varma M, Lummus Z, Bernstein D, Wymer LJ, Vesper SJ; National Exposure Research Laboratory, US Environmental Protection Agency, Cincinnati, OH 45268, USA.

[5]*J Occup Environ Med*. 2004 Jun;46(6):596-601; Quantitative polymerase chain reaction analysis of fungi in dust from homes of infants who developed idiopathic pulmonary hemorrhaging; Vesper SJ, Varma M, Wymer LJ, Dearborn DG, Sobolewski J, Haugland RA; US Environmental Protection Agency, National Exposure Research Laboratory, Cincinnati, Ohio 45268, USA. vesper.stephen@epa.gov

[6]*Damp Indoor Spaces*. The National Academy of Science. 2004: 160-162.

[7]Rosen, Gary, Ph.D., Moczik, Brad. Excerpted from *Indoor Environmental Connections*. October, 2005.

[8]Wannemacher R. W. Jr., Wiener, S. L. Trichothecene Mycotoxins. In: Zajtchuk R., Bellamy R. F., eds. *Textbook of Military Medicine: Medical Aspects of Chemical and Biologic Warfare*. Washington, DC: Office of the Surgeon General at TMM Publications, Borden Institute, Walter Reed Army Medical Center; 1997:655-77.

[9]*Food Addit Contam*. 2005 Apr; 22(4):379-88.

[10]*Arch Anim Nutr*. 2004 Aug; 58(4):311-24.

[11]*Food Chem Toxicol*. 2003 Oct; 41(10):1283-90.

[12]*Food Chem Toxicol*. 2004 May; 42(5):817-24.

[13]*Mycopathologia*. 2001; 151(3):147-53.

[14]Penicillin was discovered in 1928 by Alexander Fleming, a bacteriologist working at St. Mary's Hospital in London. He observed that a plate culture of the bacteria had been contaminated by a blue-green mold and that colonies of Staph bacteria adjacent to the mold were being dissolved. Curious, he then grew the mold as a pure culture and found that it produced a substance that killed a number of disease-causing bacteria.

[15]Caporael, L. R. (1976). "Ergotism: The Satan loosed in Salem?," *Science*, 192:21-26.

[16]Croft, W. A., Jarvis B. C., and Yatawara, C. S. 1986. "Airborne outbreak of trichothecene toxicosis." *Atmospheric Environment* 20:549-552.

[17]Hodgson, M. J., Morey, P., Leung, W., Morrow, L., Miller, D., Jarvis, B. B., Robbins, H., Halsey,

J.F., and Storey, E. 1998. "Building-associated pulmonary disease from exposure to *Stachybotrys chartarum* and *Aspergillus versicolor.*" *Journal of Occupational Environmental Medicine* 40:241-249.

[18]"Microbial Exposure and Healthy Air in Schools—Effects of Moisture Damage and Renovation," published by the Finnish National Public Health Institute (ISBN 951-740-290-2).

[19]*FEBS Lett.* 1999 Jan 8; 442(1): 89-94. Plant extracts from stinging nettle (Urtica dioica), an antirheumatic remedy, inhibit the proinflammatory transcription factor NF-kappaB; Riehemann K, Behnke B, Schulze-Osthoff K; Department of Internal Medicine I, Medical Clinics, University of Tubingen, Germany.

[20]*Food Chem Toxicol.* 2002 Aug; 40(8): 1091-7. Antitumor promoting potential of selected spice ingredients with antioxidative and anti-inflammatory activities: a short review; Surh YJ; Laboratory of Biochemistry and Molecular Toxicology, College of Pharmacy, Seoul National University, 151-742, Seoul, South Korea. surh@plaza.snu.ac.kr

APPENDIX

Moldy or Musty-smelling Basement

Keeping humidity down reduces the chances for mold to grow. Mold will not grow at less than 65% relative humidity (in the absence of water leaks)! Any groundwater, plumbing or other leaks should be fixed immediately, as part of a strategy to eliminate mold.

Mold, Mildew, Odors & Crawl Space Moisture

Mold and odors are common to crawl spaces due to the damp environment. Mold thrives in damp environments where there is plenty of food (your home) for them to eat. Sealing a crawl space floor with a thick plastic liner will prevent ground moisture from seeping into the basement, resulting in lower levels of crawl space moisture. This is the best solution to lower the relative humidity and thus prevent mold growth.

Basement Dehumidifier

A professionally installed Basement Dehumidifier will dry the air and automatically drain the water outside.

Water Leaks

Water will enter the basement through the walls, floors, and the joints between them. Over the years, contractors and engineers have developed a wide variety of sealing methods to keep basements dry. Some of these methods are more effective than others. Basements with dirt floors are particularly challenging.

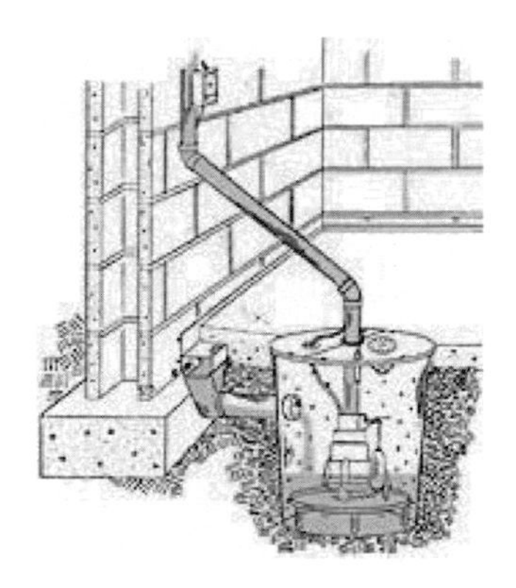

One of the best methods is to install an interior baseboard drainage system along the perimeter of the floor.

Wall Cracks and Leaks

A poured-wall crack is generally caused by concrete shrinkage. This shrinkage will continue for three years or longer after the walls are initially poured. Then, continued pressures such as soil contraction and expansion can cause further cracking and separation. So a long-term solution is needed, and one that is flexible enough to permanently fix the crack even with continued wall movement.

We recommend having a professional seal cracks with *flexible* sealant that includes a guarantee.

Hose/Water Tank Leaks

Basements are routinely flooded from sources other than ground water seepage. Leaking water heaters and washing machine hoses account for tens of thousands of flooded basements each year. One insurance industry claims specialist said, "Floods from water heater and washing machine leaks account for nearly 40% of all of our homeowner claims."

When a water heater leaks, an unlimited supply of water under pressure will flood the basement. A standard 3/8" washer hose often will shoot out up to 650 gallons per hour. If these disasters happen when nobody is home to notice, they can fill a basement up right to the top!

Several companies sell and install Water Protection Solutions to prevent these potential disasters.

Search the Internet for professionals to help you fix a problem basement by using keyword combinations of "basement," "water" and "mold."

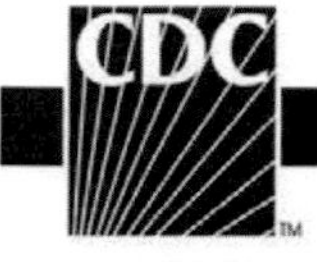

CASE DEFINITION

Trichothecene Mycotoxins

Clinical description

Trichothecene mycotoxins might be weaponized and dispersed through the air or mixed in food or beverages. Initially, route-specific effects are typically prominent. Dermal exposure leads to burning pain, redness, and blisters, and oral exposure leads to vomiting and diarrhea. Ocular exposure might result in blurred vision, and inhalational exposure might cause nasal irritation and cough. **Systemic symptoms can develop with all routes of exposure and might include weakness, ataxia, hypotension, coagulopathy, and death (1).**

Laboratory criteria for diagnosis

- *Biologic*: Selected commercial laboratories are offering immunoassays to identify trichothecenes or trichothecene-specific antibodies in human blood or urine (2, 3). However, these procedures have not been analytically validated and are not recommended.
- *Environmental*: Detection of trichothecene mycotoxins in environmental samples, as determined by FDA.

As a result of indoor air-quality investigations involving mold and potentially mold-related health effects, mycotoxin analyses of bulk environmental samples are now commercially available through environmental microbiology laboratories in the United States (4). Studies have not been done to determine the background level of trichothecenes in non-moldy homes and office buildings or nonagricultural outdoor environments. Therefore, the simple detection of trichothecenes in environmental samples does not invariably indicate an intentional contamination.

Case classification

- *Suspected*: A case in which a potentially exposed person is being evaluated by health-care workers or public health officials for poisoning by a particular chemical agent, but no specific credible threat exists.
- *Probable*: A clinically compatible case in which a high index of suspicion (credible threat or patient history regarding location and time) exists for trichothecene mycotoxins exposure, or an epidemiologic link exists between this case and a laboratory-confirmed case.
- *Confirmed*: A clinically compatible case in which laboratory tests of environmental samples have confirmed exposure.

The case can be confirmed if laboratory testing was not performed because either a predominant amount of clinical and nonspecific laboratory evidence of a particular chemical was present or a 100% certainty of the etiology of the agent is known.

Additional resources

1. Wannemacher RW Jr, Wiener SL. Trichothecene mycotoxins. In: Zajtchuk R, Bellamy RF, eds. Textbook of military medicine: medical aspects of chemical and biologic warfare. Washington, DC: Office of the Surgeon General at TMM Publications, Borden Institute, Walter Reed Army Medical Center; 1997:655-77.
2. Croft WA, Jastromski BM, Croft AL, Peters HA. Clinical confirmation of trichothecene mycotoxicosis in patient urine. J Environ Biol 2002;23:301-20.
3. Vojdani A, Thrasher HD, Madison RA, Gray MR, Heuser G, Campbell AW. Antibodies to molds and satratoxin in individuals exposed in water-damaged buildings. Arch Environ Health. 2003;58:421-32.
4. Tuomi T, Reijula K, Johnsson T, et al. Mycotoxins in crude building materials from water-damaged buildings. Appl Environ Microbiol 2000;66:1899-904.

Molds and Mycotoxins in Feedstuffs - Prevention and Treatment

L. W. Whitlow[1]
Department of Animal Science and
W. M. Hagler, Jr., Department of Poultry Science
North Carolina State University, Raleigh, NC 27695

Introduction

Molds are filamentous (fuzzy or dusty looking) fungi that occur in many feedstuffs including roughages and concentrates. Molds can infect dairy cattle, especially during stressful periods when they are immune suppressed, causing a disease referred to as a mycosis. Molds also produce poisons called mycotoxins that affect animals when they consume mycotoxin contaminated feeds. This disorder is called a mycotoxicosis. Mycotoxins are produced by a wide range of different molds and are classified as secondary metabolites meaning that their function is not essential to the mold's existence. The FAO has estimated that worldwide, about 25% of crops are affected annually with mycotoxins (Jelinek, 1987). Such surveys reveal sufficiently high occurrences and concentrations of mycotoxins to suggest that mycotoxins are a constant concern. Tables 1 and 2 provide mycotoxin occurrence and concentration of farmer submitted feedstuffs in North Carolina over several years.

Mycotoxins can be formed on crops in the field, during harvest, or during storage, processing, or feeding. Molds are present throughout the environment. The spores are high in the soil and in plant debris and lie ready to infect the growing plant in the field. Field diseases are characterized by yield loss, quality loss and mycotoxin contamination. Mold growth and the production of mycotoxins are usually associated with extremes in weather conditions leading to plant stress or hydration of feedstuffs, to poor storage practices, low feedstuff quality, and inadequate feeding conditions.

It is generally accepted that the *Aspergillus, Fusarium and Penicillium* molds are among the most important in producing mycotoxins detrimental to cattle. The major fungal genera and their mycotoxins are shown in table 3. The mycotoxins of greatest concern include: aflatoxin, which is generally produced by *Aspergillus* mold; deoxynivalenol, zearalenone, T-2 Toxin, and fumonisin, which are produced by *Fusarium* molds; and ochratoxin and PR toxin produced by *Penicillium* molds. Several other mycotoxins such as the ergots are known to affect cattle and may be prevalent at times in certain feedstuffs. There are hundreds of different mycotoxins which are diverse in their chemistry and effects on animals. It is likely that contaminated feeds will contain more than one mycotoxin. This paper is directed toward those mycotoxins thought to occur most frequently at concentrations toxic to dairy cattle. A more extensive review is available in the popular press (Whitlow and Hagler, 2004).

[1]Contact at: P. O. Box 7621, Raleigh, NC 27695-7621; Email: Lon_Whitlow@ncsu.ed

Table 1. Percentage of feeds positive for mycotoxins, in all feeds submitted by North Carolina dairy producers over a 13-year period (Whitlow et al., 1998).

	Aflatoxin n=3266	Deoxynivalenol n=5053	Zearalenone n=4563	T-2 Toxin n=5136	Fumonisin N=822
Low, range	5-19 ppb	<500 ppb	100-299 ppb	50-99ppb	<5 ppm
%	6.4	18.2	7.1	1.5	32.6
High, range	≥ 20 ppb	≥500 ppb	≥300 ppb	≥100 ppb	≥5 ppm
%	4.0	28.2	8.3	6.6	9.4
Total positive, %	10.4	46.2	15.4	8.1	42.0

n = number of samples
% = percentage of samples positive within given concentrations

Table 2. Occurrence of five mycotoxins in corn silage, corn grain and in all feed samples submitted for analysis by producers in North Carolina over a nine-year period (Whitlow et al., 1998).

	Corn Silage			Corn Grain			All Feeds		
	n	% Pos	mean ± s.d.	n	% Pos	mean ± s.d.	n	% Pos	mean ± s.d.
Aflatoxin	461	8	28 ± 19	231	9	170 ± 606	1617	7	91 ± 320
Deoxynivalenol	778	66	1991 ± 2878	362	70	1504 ± 2550	2472	58	1739 ± 1880
Zearalenone	487	30	525 ∀ 799	219	11	206 ∀ 175	1769	18	445 ± 669
T-2 toxin	717	7	569 ∀ 830	353	6	569 ∀ 690	2243	7	482 ∀ 898
Fumonisin	63	3		37	60		283	28	

n = number of samples
% = percentage of samples positive above given concentrations
mean ±s.d. = mean of the positive samples plus and minus the standard deviation

Table 3. Major toxigenic fungi and the mycotoxins thought to be the most prevalent and potentially toxic to dairy cattle.

Fungal genera	Mycotoxins
Aspergillus	Aflatoxin, Ochratoxin, Sterigmatocystin, Fumitremorgens, Fumitoxins, Fumigaclavines, Cyclopiazonoic Acid, Gliotoxin
Fusarium	Deoxynivalenol, Zearalenone, T-2 Toxin, Fumonisin, Moniliformin, Nivalenol, Diacetoxyscirpenol, Butenolide, Neosolaniol, Fusaric Acid, Fusarochromanone, Wortmannin, Fusarin C, Fusaproliferin
Penicillium	Ochratoxin, PR Toxin, Patulin, Penicillic Acid, Citrinin, Penetrem, Cyclopiazonic acid, Roquefortine, isofumigaclavines A and B, Mycophenolic acid
Claviceps	Ergot alkaloids in seed/grain of small grains, sorghum, grasses
Epichloe, and Neotyphodium	Ergot alkaloids in fescue grass.
Stachybotrys	Stachybotryotoxins, trichothecenes

Aflatoxin production by *Aspergillus flavus* in corn is favored by heat and drought stress associated with warmer climates. *Fusarium* molds commonly affect corn causing ear and stalk rots, and small grains, causing head blight (scab). In wheat, excess moisture at flowering and afterward is associated with increased incidence of mycotoxin formation. In corn, *Fusarium* diseases are more commonly associated with warm conditions at silking and with insect damage and wet conditions late in the growing season. *Penicillium* molds grow in wet and cool conditions and some require little oxygen.

Mycotoxins can increase the incidence of disease and reduce production efficiency in cattle (Coulombe, 1993; Joffe, 1986; Pier, 1992). Mycotoxins can be the primary agent causing acute health or production problems in a dairy herd, but more likely, mycotoxins are a factor contributing to chronic problems including a higher incidence of disease, poor reproductive performance or suboptimal milk production. They exert their effects through four primary mechanisms: (1) intake reduction or feed refusal, (2) reduced nutrient absorption and impaired metabolism; (3) alterations in the endocrine and exocrine systems; and (4) suppression of the immune system. Recognition of the impact of mycotoxins on animal production has been limited by the difficulty of diagnosis. Symptoms are often nonspecific and the result of a progression of effects, making a diagnosis difficult or impossible because of the complex clinical results with a wide diversity of symptoms. The difficulty of diagnosis is increased due to limited research, occurrence of multiple mycotoxins, non-uniform distribution, interactions with other factors, and problems of sampling and analysis.

Because of the difficulty of diagnosis, the determination of a mycotoxin problem becomes a process of elimination and association. Certain basics can be helpful: 1)

Mycotoxins should be considered as a possible primary factor resulting in production losses and increased incidence of disease. 2) Documented symptoms in ruminants or other species can be used as a general guide to symptoms observed in the field. 3) Systemic effects as well as specific damage to target tissues can be used as a guide to possible causes. 4) Post mortem examinations may indicate no more than gut irritation, edema or generalized tissue inflammation. 5) Because of the immune suppressing effects of mycotoxins, atypical diseases or increased incidence of disease may be observed. 6) Responses to added dietary sorbents or dilution of the contaminated feed may help in diagnosis. 7) Feed analyses should be performed, but accurate sampling is a problem (Schiefer, 1990).

Symptoms of a mycotoxicosis in a dairy herd vary depending on the mycotoxins involved and their interactions with other stress factors. The more stressed cows, such as fresh cows, are most affected, perhaps because their immune systems are already suppressed. Symptoms of mycotoxins may be nonspecific and wide ranging. Symptoms may be few or many. Symptoms may include: reduced production, reduced feed consumption, intermittent diarrhea (sometimes with bloody or dark manure), reduced feed intake, unthriftiness, rough hair coat, reduced reproductive performance including irregular estrus cycles, embryonic mortalities, pregnant cows showing estrus, and decreased conception rates. There generally is an increase in incidence of disease, such as displaced abomasum, ketosis, retained placenta, metritis, mastitis, and fatty livers. Cows do not respond well to veterinary therapy.

Molds can cause disease

A mold (fungal) infection resulting in disease is referred to as a mycosis. Fungal pathogens include *Aspergillus fumigatus, Candida albicans, Candida vaginitis* and certain species of *Fusarium*.

Aspergillus fumigatus has been proposed as the pathogenic agent associated with mycotic hemorrhagic bowel syndrome (HBS) in dairy cattle (Puntenney et al., 2003). *A. fumigatus* is thought to be a fairly common mold in both hay (Shadmi et al., 1974) and silage (Cole et al., 1977). While healthy cows with an active immune system are more resistant to mycotic infections, dairy cows in early lactation are immune suppressed (Kehrli et al., 1989a&b) and HBS is more likely in fresh cows (Puntenney et al., 2003). It is theorized that in a mycosis, mycotoxins produced by the invading fungi can suppress immunity, therefore increasing the infectivity of the fungus. *A. fumigatus* produces a mycotoxin, gliotoxin, which is an immune suppressant. Gliotoxin has been present in animals infected with *A. fumigatus* (Bauer et al., 1989). Reeves et al. (2004) using an insect model demonstrated the significance of gliotoxin in increasing the virulence of *A. fumigatus*. Niyo et al. (1988a, b) have demonstrated that in rabbits, T-2 toxin decreased phagocytosis of *A. fumigatus* conidia by alveolar macrophages and increased severity of experimental aspergillosis. It is possible that gliotoxin, T-2 toxin or other mycotoxins that suppress immunity may be a trigger to increased infectivity by the fungus, ultimately resulting in HBS or other fungal infections. If this is true, then reducing animal exposure to mycotoxins may be a key to control of mycoses such as HBS. A commercial feed additive with anti-fungal and adsorbent properties appears to reduce HBS (Puntenney et al., 2003), although these additives can have other functions including the reduction of mold growth.

Toxicity of Individual Mycotoxins

Aflatoxin

Aflatoxins are a family of extremely toxic, mutagenic, and carcinogenic compounds produced by *Aspergillus flavus* and *A. parasiticus* (Deiner et al., 1987; Kurtzman et al., 1987). Toxigenic *A. flavus* isolates produce aflatoxins B1, and B2 and toxigenic *A. parasiticus* isolates produce aflatoxins B1, B2, G1, and G2 (Cotty et al., 1994). Aflatoxin B1 is a carcinogen and is excreted in milk in the form of aflatoxin M1. Table 4 provides the Food and Drug Administration (FDA) action levels for aflatoxin in feeds and milk. The FDA limits aflatoxin to no more than 20 ppb in lactating dairy feeds and to 0.5 ppb in milk. A thumb rule is that milk aflatoxin concentrations equal about 1.7% of the aflatoxin concentration in the total ration dry matter. Cows consuming diets containing 30 ppb aflatoxin can produce milk containing aflatoxin residues above the FDA action level of 0.5 ppb. In Europe the regulatory levels of aflatoxin are 20 ppb for dairy feeds and 0.05 ppb in milk, therefore, an illegal milk residue can occur when feed contains more than 3 ppb of aflatoxin. Figure 1 shows the clearance and appearance of aflatoxin in milk over a 16 day period in association with the feeding of clean or aflatoxin-contaminated corn, in diets with and without clay products added at 1%.

Table 4. U.S. Food and Drug Administration action levels for total aflatoxins in food and feed[a]

Food or Feedstuff	Concentration (ppb)
All products, except milk, designated for humans	20
Corn for immature animals and dairy cattle	20
Corn and peanut products for breeding beef cattle, swine, and mature poultry	100
Corn and peanut products for finishing swine (>100 lb)	200
Corn and peanut products for finishing beef cattle	300
Cottonseed meal (as a feed ingredient)	300
All other feedstuffs	20
Milk[b]	0.5

[a] Wood and Trucksess, 1998. [b] Aflatoxin M1.

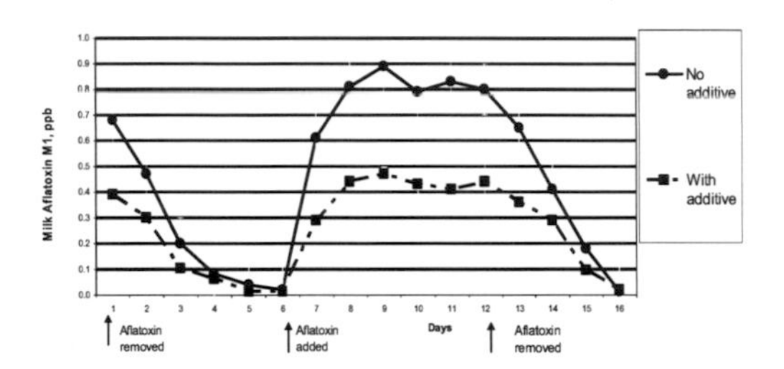

Figure 1. Concentration of aflatoxin M1 in milk of dairy cows over a 16 day period associated with consumption of aflatoxin-contaminated or clean corn in diets with and without clay products added at 1% of the diets. Milk aflatoxin concentrations are reduced by dietary addition of clay products. Appearance and clearance of aflatoxin in milk are rapid and unaffected by dietary clay additions. Diaz et al., 2004.

Symptoms of acute aflatoxicosis in mammals include: inappetance, lethargy, ataxia, rough hair coat, and pale, enlarged fatty livers. Symptoms of chronic aflatoxin exposure include reduced feed efficiency and milk production, jaundice, and decreased appetite (Nibbelink, 1986). Aflatoxin lowers resistance to diseases and interferes with vaccine-induced immunity in livestock (Diekman and Green, 1992). In beef cattle, Garrett et al. (1968) showed an effect on weight gain and intake with diets containing 700 ppb aflatoxin, but if increases in liver weights are used as the criteria for toxicity, 100 ppb would be considered toxic to beef cattle. Production and health of dairy herds may be affected at dietary aflatoxin levels above 100 ppb which is considerably higher than the amount that produces illegal milk residues (Patterson and Anderson 1982 and Masri et al. 1969). Guthrie (1979) showed when lactating dairy cattle in a field situation were consuming 120 ppb aflatoxin reproductive efficiency declined and when cows were changed to an aflatoxin free diet, milk production increased over 25%. Applebaum et al. (1982) showed that impure aflatoxin produced by culture reduced production while equal amounts of pure aflatoxin did not.

Aflatoxin is more often found in corn, peanuts and cottonseed grown in warm and humid climates. Aflatoxin can be found in more temperate areas in some years as was seen in the drought year of 1988 when aflatoxin was found in 5% of corn grain in the Midwestern U.S. (Russell, et al., 1991). The General Accounting Office (GAO, 1991) concluded that industry, federal and state programs are effective in detecting and controlling aflatoxin and that it is doubtful that additional programs or limits would reduce the risk of aflatoxin in the food supply.

Deoxynivalenol (DON) or Vomitoxin

Deoxynivalenol is a *Fusarium* produced mycotoxin that is one of the most commonly detected in feed. It is sometimes called vomitoxin because it was first associated with vomiting in swine. Surveys have shown DON to be a primary mycotoxin associated with swine disorders including feed refusals, diarrhea, emesis, reproductive failure, and deaths. The impact of DON on dairy cattle is not established, but clinical data show an association between DON contamination of diets and poor performance in dairy herds, but without establishing a cause and effect (Whitlow et al., 1994). Dairy cattle consuming diets contaminated primarily with DON (2.5 ppm) have responded favorably (1.5 kg milk, P<.05) to the dietary inclusion of mycotoxin binders, providing circumstantial evidence that DON reduces milk production (Diaz, et al., 2001). Field reports help substantiate an association of DON with poor performing dairy herds (Gotlieb, 1997 and Seglar, 1997). Results from a Canadian study using 18 first-lactation cows during mid-lactation (average 19.5 kg milk), showed that cows consuming DON contaminated diets (2.6 to 6.5 ppm) tended (P<0.16) to produce less milk (13% or 1.4 kg) than did cows consuming clean feed (Charmley et al., 1993). DON had no effect on milk production in 8 cows fed over a 21 day period (Ingalls, 1994). Beef cattle and sheep have tolerated up to 21 ppm of dietary DON without obvious effects (DiCostanzo et al., 1995).

Like other mycotoxins, pure DON added to diets, does not have as much toxicity as does DON supplied from naturally contaminated feeds (Foster et al., 1986). This is thought to result from the interaction of multiple mycotoxins in naturally contaminated feeds. These mycotoxins can interact to cause symptoms that are different or more severe than expected. For example, it is now known that fusaric acid interacts with DON to cause the vomiting effects earlier attributed to DON alone and resulted in use of the trivial name of vomitoxin for DON (Smith and MacDonald, 1991). It is believed that DON serves as a marker, indicating that feed was exposed to a situation conducive for mold growth and possible formation of several mycotoxins. FDA's advisory levels are in table 5.

Table 5. U.S. Food and Drug Administration advisory levels for deoxynivalenol in wheat and wheat derived products[a]

Product	Concentration, ppm
All finished wheat products, e.g. flour, bran and germ, for human consumption	1
Grains and grain by-products destined for ruminating beef cattle and cattle and cattle in feedlots older than 4 months and for chickens (these ingredients should not exceed 50% of the diet)	10
Grains and grain by-products destined for swine (these ingredients should not exceed 20% of the diet)	5
Grains and grain by-products for all other animals (these ingredients should not exceed 40% of the diet)	5

[a]Wood and Trucksess, 1998

T-2 Toxin (T-2)

T-2 toxin is a very potent *Fusarium* produced mycotoxin that occurs in a low proportion of feed samples (<10%). Russell, et al. (1991) found 13% of Midwestern corn grain contaminated with T-2 toxin in a survey of the 1988 drought damaged crop.

T-2 is associated with reduced feed consumption, loss in yield, gastroenteritis, intestinal hemorrhage, reduced reproductive performance and death. Effects are less well established in cattle than in laboratory animals (Wannemacher et al., 1991). T-2 toxin is associated with gastroenteritis, intestinal hemorrhages (Petrie et al., 1977; Mirocha et al., 1976) and death (Hsu et al., 1972 and Kosuri et al., 1970). Dietary T-2 toxin at 640 ppb for 20 days resulted in bloody feces, enteritis, abomasal and ruminal ulcers and death (Pier et al., 1980). Weaver et al. (1980) showed that T-2 was associated with feed refusal and gastrointestinal lesions in a cow, but did not show a hemorrhagic syndrome. Kegl and Vanyi (1991) observed bloody diarrhea, low feed consumption, decreased milk production and absence of estrus cycles in cows exposed to T-2. Serum immunoglobulins and complement proteins were lowered in calves receiving T-2 toxin (Mann et al., 1983). Gentry et al. (1984) demonstrated a reduction in white blood cell and neutrophil counts in calves. McLaughlin et al. (1977) demonstrated that primary basis of T-2 reduced immunity is reduced protein synthesis.

Zearalenone (ZEA)

Zearalenone is a *Fusarium* produced mycotoxin that has a chemical structure similar to estrogen and can produce an estrogenic response in animals. Zearalenone is associated with ear and stalk rots in corn and with scab in wheat (Christensen et al., 1988).

Controlled studies with ZEA at high levels have failed to reproduce the degree of toxicity that has been associated with zearalenone contaminated feeds in field observations. A controlled study with non-lactating cows fed up to 500 mg of ZEA (calculated dietary concentrations of about 25 ppm ZEA) showed no obvious effects except that corpora lutea were smaller in treated cows (Weaver et al., 1986b). In a similar study with heifers receiving 250 mg of ZEA by gelatin capsule (calculated dietary concentrations of about 25 ppm ZEA), conception rate was depressed about 25%; otherwise, no obvious effects were noted (Weaver et al., 1986a).

Several case reports have related ZEA to estrogenic responses in ruminants including abortions (Kellela and Ettala, 1984; Khamis et al., 1986; Mirocha et al., 1968; Mirocha et al., 1974; Roine et al., 1971). Symptoms have included vaginitis, vaginal secretions, poor reproductive performance and mammary gland enlargement of virgin heifers. In a field study (Coppock et al., 1990), diets with about 660 ppb ZEA and 440 ppb DON resulted in poor consumption, depressed milk production, diarrhea, increase in reproductive tract infections, and total reproductive failure.

New Zealand workers (Towers, et al., 1995) have measured blood ZEA and metabolites ("zearalenone") to estimate ZEA intake. Dairy herds with low fertility had higher levels of blood "zearalenone". Individual cows within herds examined by palpation and determined to be cycling had lower blood "zearalenone" levels than did cows that were not cycling. The reproductive problems in dairy cattle were associated with dietary ZEA concentrations of about 400 ppb.

Fumonisin (FB)

Fumonisin B_1 produced by *F. verticillioides*, was first isolated in 1988. It causes leucoencephalomalacia in horses, pulmonary edema in swine and hepatoxicity in rats. It is carcinogenic in rats and mice (NTP, 1999) and is thought to be a promoter of esophageal cancer in humans (Chu and Li, 1994; Rheeder et al., 1992). Fumonisins are structurally similar to sphingosine, a component of sphingolipids, which are in high concentrations in certain nerve tissues such as myelin. Fumonisin toxicity results from blockage of sphingolipid biosynthesis and thus degeneration of tissues rich in sphingolipids.

While FB_1 is much less potent in ruminants than in hogs, it has now been shown toxic to sheep, goats, beef cattle, and dairy cattle. Osweiler et al. (1993) fed 18 young steers either 15, 31 or 148 ppm of fumonisin in a short term study (31 days). With the highest feeding level, there were mild liver lesions found in two of six calves, and the group had elevated liver enzymes indicative of liver damage. Lymphocyte blastogenesis was significantly impaired at the end of the feeding period in the group having the highest dose.

Dairy cattle (Holsteins and Jerseys) fed diets containing 100 ppm fumonisin for approximately 7 days prior to freshening and for 70 days thereafter demonstrated lower milk production (6 kg/cow/day), explained primarily by reduced feed consumption (Figure 2, Diaz et al., 2000). Increases in serum enzymes concentrations suggested mild liver disease. Because of greater production stress, dairy cattle may be more sensitive to fumonisin than are beef cattle. Fumonisin carryover from feed to milk is thought to be negligible (Scott et al., 1994).

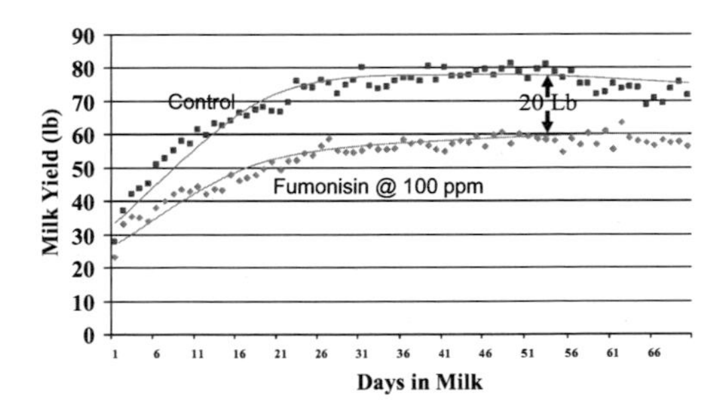

Figure 2. Daily milk production (31.2 vs 24.2, P ≤ .05) for dairy cows n = 26 (Holsteins and Jerseys) consuming control diets (< 1 ppm fumonisin) or fumonisin-contaminated diets (100 ppm fumonisin) respectively for about 7 days prior to parturition and for 70 days in lactation. Diaz et al. 2000.

A USDA, APHIS survey of 1995 corn from Missouri, Iowa and Illinois found that 6.9% contained more than 5 ppm fumonisin B1 (Anon, 1995). Fumonisin was prevalent in Midwestern corn from the wet 1993 season. Corn screenings contain about 10 times the fumonisin content of the original corn.

Table 6 gives the FDA's guidance for industry on fumonisin levels in human foods and animal feeds.

Table 6. U.S. Food and Drug Administration Guidance for Industry on Fumonisin Levels in Human Foods and Animal Feeds[a]

	Total Fumonisins (FB_1+FB_2+FB_3) Concentration (ppm)
Human Foods	
Product	
Degermed dry milled corn products (e.g., flaking grits, corn grits, corn meal, corn flour with fat content of < 2.25%, dry weight basis)	2
Whole or partially degermed dry milled corn products (e.g., flaking grits, corn grits, corn meal, corn flour with fat content of $\geq$ 2.25 %, dry weight basis)	4
Dry milled corn bran	4
Cleaned corn intended for masa production	4
Cleaned corn intended for popcorn	3
Animal Feeds	
Corn and corn by-products intended for:	
Equids and rabbits (no more than 20% of diet)[b]	5
Swine and catfish (no more than 50% of diet)[b]	20
Breeding ruminants, breeding poultry and breeding mink and including lactating dairy cattle and hens laying eggs for human consumption (no more than 50% of diet)[b]	30
Ruminants $\geq$ 3 months old being raised for slaughter and mink being raised for pelt production (no more than 50% of diet)[b]	60
Poultry being raised for slaughter (no more than 50% of diet)[b]	100
All other species or classes of livestock and pet animals (no more than 50% of diet)[b]	10

[a] Federal Register, 2001. [b] Limits on ingredients are on a dry weight basis

Other Mycotoxins

In 2001, the FDA released a guidance document for fumonisin in human foods and animal feeds. It is recommended that human food products should contain no more than 2 to 4 ppm of total fumonisins. For dairy cattle, the guideline recommends that contaminated corn or corn-byproducts be limited to no more than 50% of the diet, and that the maximum concentrations of total fumonisins in corn and corn by-products are 30 ppm for lactating and breeding age cattle and no more that 10 ppm for calves (Federal Register, 2001). Because fumonisin is associated with reduced feed consumption, there is a concern that low levels of fumonisin interacting with other mycotoxins may reduce milk production.

Many other mycotoxins may affect ruminants but they are thought to occur less frequently or be less potent. Diacetoxyscirpenol, HT-2 and neosolaniol may occur along with T-2 toxin and cause similar symptoms. Ochratoxin has been reported to affect cattle, but it is rapidly degraded in the rumen and thus thought to be of little consequence except for pre-ruminants. Tremorgens such as fumigaclavine A and B produced by *Aspergillus fumigatus* are thought to be common in silages of the southeastern US and were toxic to beef cattle in a field case in Georgia (Cole, et al., 1977). Tremorgens can cause anorexia, diarrhea, unthriftiness and irritability. Mycotoxins such as rubratoxin, citrinin, patulin, cyclopiazonic acid, sterigmatocystin and ergot alkaloids may also be of importance. Mycotoxins in forages have been reviewed by Lacey (1991).

Mycotoxin Testing

Analytical techniques for mycotoxins are improving. Several commercial laboratories are available and provide screens for a large array of mycotoxins. Cost of analyses has been a constraint but can be insignificant compared with the economic consequences of production and health losses related to mycotoxin contamination. Newer immunoassays have reduced the cost of analyses.

Collection of representative feed samples is a problem primarily because molds can produce very large amounts of mycotoxins in small areas making the mycotoxin level highly variable within the lot of feed (Whittaker et al., 1991). Core sampling of horizontal silos shows mycotoxins can be highly variable throughout the silo. Because mycotoxins can form in the collected sample, samples should be preserved and delivered to the lab quickly. Samples can be dried, frozen or treated with a mold inhibitor before shipping.

Concentrations of mycotoxins, that are considered as acceptable and of no consequence, should be conservatively low due to non-uniform distribution, uncertainties in sampling and analysis, the potential for multiple sources in the diet, and interacting factors affecting toxicity (Hamilton, 1984).

Prevention and Treatment

Prevention of mycotoxin formation is essential since there are few ways to completely overcome problems once mycotoxins are present. Drought and insect damage are most important in instigating molding and mycotoxin formation in the field. Choosing varieties that have some resistance to fungal disease, and resistance to insect damage (Bt hybrids) have fewer field produced mycotoxins. Varieties should be adapted to the growing area. Irrigation can reduce mycotoxin formation in the field. When harvesting, avoid lodged or fallen material, because contact with soil can increase mycotoxins. Mycotoxins increase with delayed harvest, and with late season rain and cool periods. Damaged grains have increased mycotoxin levels, thus for dry grain storage, harvesting equipment should be maintained to avoid kernel damage. Mycotoxin concentrations are greatest in the fines, and in broken and damaged kernels, thus cleaning can greatly reduce mycotoxin concentrations in the feedstuff. After harvest, grains should not be allowed to remain at levels of moisture greater than 15 to 18%. While there is little mold growth in grain at moisture levels below 15%, drying to levels below 14% and preferably to <13% help to compensate for non-uniform moisture concentrations throughout the grain mass. The high ambient temperatures of Florida also dictate that grain must be dried to the lower levels because higher temperatures increase the amount of free moisture (water activity) in the grain which is the primary cause of mold growth in storage. Storage should be sufficient to eliminate moisture migration, moisture condensation or leaks. Grain stored for more than two weeks should be kept aerated and cool. Aeration is important because as molds start to grow in isolated spots, the moisture produced by metabolism is sufficient to stimulate spread of the mold growth. Aeration reduces moisture migration and non-uniform moisture concentrations. Commodity sheds should protect feedstuffs from rain or other water sources. They should be constructed with a vapor barrier in the floor to reduce moisture. If wet feeds are stored in commodity sheds near dry feeds, a method must be devised to prevent moisture contamination of the dry feed. Bins, silos and other storage facilities should be cleaned to eliminate source of inoculation. Check stored feed at intervals to determine if heating and molding are occurring. Organic acids can be used as preservatives for feeds too high in moisture for proper storage. Table 7 gives recommendations on use of propionic acid for preservation of grain.

Table 7. Recommended Application Rates for Pure Propionic Acid for the Preservation of High-Moisture Grains not Stored in a Silo

Grain Moisture	Amount of acid per ton of grain for storage length of: 6 Mo.	2 Mo.
%	lb	lb
25	12	15
30	16	20
35	17	25
40	20	30

It can be difficult to make hay at moisture levels low enough to prevent mold growth. Mold will grow in hay at moisture levels above 12 to 15%. As molds and other microorganisms grow they produce heat and cause deterioration. Heating can become so intense as to cause spontaneous combustion and hay fires. Feeding moldy hay can reduce intake and performance and the deterioration results in reduced nutritional value. Hay harvested at high moistures will tend to equilibrate to moisture contents of 12 to 14%, but rate of moisture loss is dependent on moisture at harvest, air movement, humidity, air temperature, bale density and the storage facility. Rate of dry down is enhanced by ventilation, creation of air spaces between bales, reduced size of stacks, alternation in the direction of stacking and avoidance of other wet products in the same area.

Prevention of mycotoxins in silage includes following accepted silage making practices aimed at preventing deterioration primarily by quickly reducing pH and elimination of oxygen. Generally accepted silage making practices are to harvest at the proper moisture content; chop uniformly at the proper length, fill the silo rapidly; pack the silage sufficiently; use an effective fermentation aide; and cover completely and well. Infiltration of air after ensiling can allow growth of acid tolerant microorganisms, an increase in the pH and then mold growth. *Penicillium* molds are somewhat acid tolerant and may grow if any air is present. Some additives are beneficial in reducing pH very rapidly and therefore they can reduce mold growth and mycotoxin formation. Ammonia, propionic acid, sorbic acid and microbial or enzymatic silage additives are shown to be at least partially effective at inhibiting mold growth. Ammonia may prevent silage from reaching a low pH, but it can reduce mold growth through direct inhibition of the mold. Organic acids provide the acidity for preservation without relying solely on acids produced in the ensiling process. Organic acids may be used to treat the entire silage mass, or to selectively treat the outer layers of the silo. Organic acids are also used during feedout to treat the silo feeding face and/or the TMR in an effort to reduce continuous deterioration of the feeding face and to reduce heating in the feed bunk. Silo size should be matched to herd size to insure daily removal of silage at a rate faster than deterioration. In warm climates it is best to remove a foot of silage daily from the feeding face. The feeding face of silos should be cleanly cut and disturbed as little as possible to prevent aeration into the silage mass. Silage or other wet feeds should be fed immediately after storage removal. Spoilage should not be fed and feed bunks should be cleaned regularly.

As with silage, high moisture grains or byproduct feeds must be stored at proper moisture contents in a well maintained structure and managed well to prevent mold. Wet feeds must be handled in quantities which allow them to be fed out within 7 to 10 days. Organic acids are very helpful in preventing mold in wet commodity feeds and can extend storage life. Discard any spoilage.

Obviously moldy feed should be avoided. Spoilage or deteriorated silage can reduce feed consumption, fiber digestibility and production. If unacceptably high levels of mycotoxins occur, dilution or removal of the contaminated feed is preferable; however, it is often impossible to completely replace some feeds in the ration, particularly the forage ingredients. Ammoniation of grains can destroy some mycotoxins, but there is no practical method to detoxify affected forages. Cleaning grains can be helpful. Dietary strategies to counteract the effects of mycotoxins have been reviewed (Galvano et al., 2001). Increasing dietary levels of nutrients such as protein, energy and antioxidants may be advisable. Animals exposed to aflatoxin show marginal responses to increased protein. In some situations, poultry respond to water soluble vitamins or to specific minerals. Acidic diets seem to exacerbate effects of mycotoxins, and therefore adequate dietary fiber and buffers are recommended. Because mycotoxins reduce feed consumption, feeding management to encourage intake can be helpful. Dry cows, springing heifers and calves should receive the cleanest feed possible. Transition rations can reduce stress in fresh cows. Strategic use of mold inhibitors can be beneficial.

When animals are exposed to mycotoxins, favorable results have been seen when absorbent materials such as clays (bentonites and others), complex indigestible carbohydrates such as glucomannans or mannanoligiosaccharides, and other similar products are added to mycotoxin contaminated diets of rats, poultry, swine and cattle. Some of these products have been reviewed by Huwig et al., (2001), and yet many studies with good results have been published since this review. Responses in dairy cattle to some of these products have been very encouraging. Overall results are variable by type and amount of binder, specific mycotoxins and their amounts, animal species, and interactions of other dietary ingredients. No adsorbent product is approved by the FDA for the prevention or treatment of mycotoxicoses. Several of these adsorbent materials are recognized as safe feed additives (GRAS) and are used in diets for other purposes such as flow agents, pellet binders, etc. Figure 3 shows the effects of some feed additives on reducing aflatoxin in milk, theoretically as a result of binding the aflatoxin and therefore reducing intestinal absorption.

Summary

Mycotoxins are prevalent in feedstuffs.
Many different mycotoxins exist.
Mycotoxins affect dairy cattle in many ways, and the most important is perhaps immunosuppression.
While mycotoxins can cause acute toxicity, they are more likely to cause chronic problems of increased disease and decreased milk production.
Diagnosis of a mycotoxicosis is difficult and indirect, but mycotoxins should be considered as a potential cause of increased disease and loss of production.
Contamination of milk by aflatoxin can cause huge economic losses. Management of crops and feeds is important to reduce mycotoxin contamination. Certain feed additives are proved to be helpful in treatment.

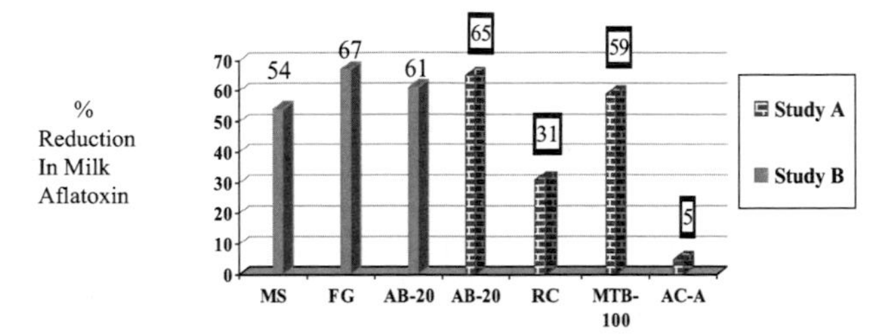

Figure 3. Effect of feed additives on reduction of milk aflatoxin residues in two studies. **MS,** mycrosorb, a sodium bentonite fed at 1% of DM (American Colliod Co.) FG, flowguard, a sodium bentonite fed at 1% of DM intake (La Port Biochem.), **AB-20**, a sodium bentonite fed at 1% of DM intake (Prince AgriProducts, Inc.). **RC**, Red Crown, a calcium bentonite fed at 1% of DM intake (Prince AgriProducts, Inc.) and **MTB-100**, a modified glucomannan product fed at 0.05% of DM intake (Alltech, Inc.) significantly reduced ($P < .0001$) AFM1 residues in milk. **AC-A**, an activated charcoal fed at 0.25% of DM intake had no effect. Diaz, et al. 2004. Mycopathologia 157:233-241.

Areas of Needed Information

CAST (2003) published a list of major needs for research, which included: surveillance of feeds for mycotoxin presence and quantity; assessment of control methods for prevention and treatment; development of resistant plants; improvement of sampling and analysis; improved understanding of effects on animals particularly on immunosuppression; toxicological evaluation of newly discovered mycotoxins and assessment of economic effects.

References

Anonymous, 1995. USDA. APHIS. "Mycotoxin Levels in the 1995 Midwest Preharvest Corn Crop". Veterinary Services Factsheet N195.1295. The National Veterinary Services Laboratory, Ames, Iowa.

Applebaum, R.S., R.E. Brackett, D.W. Wiseman, and E.L. Marth. 1982. Responses of dairy cows to dietary aflatoxin: feed intake and yield, toxin content, and quality of milk of cows treated with pure and impure aflatoxin. J. Dairy Sci. 65:1503-1508.

Bauer, J., A. Gareis, A. Gott, and B. Gedek. 1989. Isolation of a mycotoxin (gliotoxin) from a bovine udder infected with *Aspergillus fumigatus*. J Med Vet Mycol 27:45–50.

CAST, Council for Agricultural Science and Technology. 2003. "Mycotoxins: Risks in Plant Animal and Human Systems". Task Force Report No. 139. Ames, Iowa.

Charmley, E., H.L. Trenholm, B.K. Thompson, D. Vudathala, J.W.G. Nicholson, D.B. Prelusky and L.L. Charmley. 1993. Influence of level of deoxynivalenol in the diet of dairy cows on feed intake, milk production and its composition. J. Dairy Sci. 6:3580-3587.

Chu, F.S., and G.Y. Li. 1994. Simultaneous occurrence of fumonisin B 1 and other mycotoxins in moldy corn collected from the People's Republic of China in regions with high incidences of esophageal cancer. Appl. Environ. Microbiol. 60:847-852.

Christensen, C.M., C.J. Mirocha, and R.A. Meronuck. 1988. "Molds and Mycotoxins in Feeds". Minn. Ext. Serv. Bull. AG-FO-3538. Univ. MN, St. Paul.

Cole, R.J., J.W. Kirksey, J.W. Dorner, D.M. Wilson, J.C. Johnson, Jr., A.N. Johnson, D.M. Bedell, J.P. Springer, K.K. Chexal, J.C. Clardy, and R.H. Cox. 1977. Mycotoxins produced by *Aspergillus fumigatus* species isolated from moldy silage. J. Agric. Food Chem. 25:826-830.

Coppock, R.W., M.S. Mostrom, C.G. Sparling, B. Jacobsen, and S.C. Ross. 1990. Apparent zearalenone intoxication in a dairy herd from feeding spoiled acid-treated corn. Vet. Hum. Toxicol. 32:246-248.

Cotty, P.J ., P. Bayman, D.S. Egel, and D.S. Elias. 1994. Agriculture, aflatoxins and *Aspergillus*. pp. 1-27. In: K.A. Powell, A. Fenwick and J.F. Peberdy (Eds) "The Genus *Aspergillus*" Plenum Press. New York.

Coulombe, R.A. 1993. Symposium: biological action of mycotoxins. J. Dairy Sci. 76:880-891.

Deiner, U.L., R.J. Cole, T.H Sanders, G.A. Payne, L.S. Lee, and M.A. Klich. 1987. Epidemiology of aflatoxin formation by *Aspergillus flavus*. Ann. Rev. Phytopathology 25:240-270.

Diaz, D.E., W.M. Hagler, Jr., J.T. Blackwelder, J.A. Eve, B.A. Hopkins, K.L. Anderson, F.T. Jones, and L.W. Whitlow. 2004. Aflatoxin binders II: reduction of aflatoxin M1 in milk by sequestering agents of cows consuming aflatoxin in feed. Mycopathologia 157: 233-241.

Diaz, D.E., W. M. Hagler, Jr., B.A. Hopkins, R.A. Patton, C. Brownie, and L.W. Whitlow. 2001. The effect of inclusion of a clay type sequestering agent on milk production of dairy cattle consuming mycotoxins contaminated feeds. J. Dairy Sci. 84(abstr.):1554.

Diaz, D.E., B.A. Hopkins, L.M. Leonard, W.M. Hagler, Jr., and L.W. Whitlow. 2000. Effect of fumonisin on lactating dairy cattle. J. Dairy Sci. 83(abstr.):1171.

DiCostanzo, A., L. Johnston, H. Windels, and M. Murphy. 1995. A review of the effects of molds and mycotoxins in ruminants. Professional Animal Scientist 12:138-150.

Diekman, D.A., and M.L. Green. 1992. Mycotoxins and reproduction in domestic livestock. J. Anim. Sci. 70:1615-1627.

Federal Register, 2001. Guidance for industry: Fumonisin levels in human foods and animal feeds. Federal Register 66(No.218, November 9, 2001):56688-56689.

Foster, B.C., H.L. Trenholm, D.W. Friend, B.K. Thompson, and K.E. Hartin. 1986. Evaluation of different sources of deoxynivalenol (vomitoxin) fed to swine. Can. J. Anim. Sci. 66:1149-1154.

Galvano, F., A. Piva, A. Ritieni, and G. Galvano. 2001. Dietary strategies to counteract the effects of mycotoxins: A review. J Food Prot. 64:120–131.

GAO. 1991. Food safety and quality. Existing detection and control programs minimize aflatoxin. Report RCED-91-109.

Garrett, W.N., H. Heitman, Jr., and A.N. Booth. 1968, Aflatoxin toxicity in beef cattle.

Proc. Soc. Exp. Biol. Med. 127:188-190.
Gentry, P.A., M.L. Ross, and P.K-C. Chan. 1984. Effect of T-2 toxin on bovine hematological and serum enzyme parameters. Vet. Hum. Toxicol. 26:24-24.
Gotlieb, A. 1997. Causes of mycotoxins in silages. pp. 213-221. In: "Silage: Field to Feedbunk", NRAES-99, Northeast Regional Agricultural Engineering Service, Ithaca, NY.
Guthrie, L.D. 1979. Effects of Aflatoxin in corn on production and reproduction in dairy cattle. J Dairy Sci. 62 (abstr.):134.
Hamilton, P.B. 1984. Determining safe levels of mycotoxins. J. Food Prot. 47:570-575.
Joffe, A.Z. 1986. "*Fusarium* Species: Their Biology and Toxicology". John Wiley and Sons, Inc., New York.
Hsu, I.C., C.B. Smalley, F.M. Strong, and W.E. Ribelin. 1972. Identification of T-2 toxin in moldy corn associated with a lethal toxicosis in dairy cattle. Appl. Microbiol. 24:684-690.
Huwig, A., S. Freimund, O. Kappeli, and H. Dutler. 2001. Mycotoxin detoxication of animal feed by different adsorbents. Toxicol. Lett. 122:179–188.
Ingalls, J.R. 1996. Influence of deoxynivalenol on feed consumption by dairy cows. Anim. Feed Sci. Tech. 60:297-300.
Jelinek, C.F. 1987. Distribution of mycotoxin - An analysis of worldwide commodities data, including data from FAO/WHO/UNEP food contamination monitoring programme. Joint FAO/WHO/UNEP Second International Conference on Mycotoxins. Bangkok, Thailand, September 28 to October 3, 1987.
Kallela, K., and E. Ettala. 1984. The oestrogenic *Fusarium* toxin (zearalenone) in hay as a cause of early abortions in the cow. Nord. Vet. Med. 36:305-309.
Kegl, T., and A. Vanyi. 1991. T-2 fusariotoxicosis in a cattle stock. Magyar Allatorvosok Lapja 46:467-471.
Kehrli, M.E., Jr., B.J. Nonnecke, and J.A. Roth. 1989a. Alterations in bovine lymphocyte function during the periparturient period. Am. J. Vet. Res. 50:215.
Kehrli, M.E., Jr., B.J. Nonnecke, and J.A. Roth. 1989b. Alterations in bovine neutrophil function during the periparturient period. Am. J. Vet. Res. 50:207.
Khamis, Y., H.A. Hammad, and N.A. Hemeida. 1986. Mycotoxicosis with oestrogenic effect in cattle. Zuchthyg. 21:233-236.
Kosuri, N.R., M.D. Grave, S.G. Yates, W.H. Tallent, J.J. Ellis, I.A. Wolff, and R.E. Nichols. 1970. Response of cattle to mycotoxins of *Fusarium tricinctum* isolated from corn and fescue. J. Am. Vet. Med. Assoc. 157:938-940.
Kurtzman, C.P., B.W. Horn, and C.W. Hesseltine. 1987. *Aspergillus* nomius, a new aflatoxin-producing species related to *Aspergillus flavus* and *Aspergillus tamarii*. Antonie van Leeuwenhoek 53:147-158.
Lacey, J. 1991. Natural occurrence of mycotoxins in growing and conserved forage crops. pp. 363-397. In: J. E. Smith and R. E. Henderson (Eds.), "Mycotoxins and Animal Foods". CRC Press, Boca Raton.
Mann, D.D., G.M. Buening, B. Hook, and G.D. Osweiler. 1983. Effects of T-2 mycotoxin on bovine serum proteins. J. Am. Vet. Med. Assoc. 44:1757-1759.
Masri, M.S., V.C. Garcia, and J.R. Page. 1969. The aflatoxin M_1 content of milk from cows fed known amounts of aflatoxin. Vet. Rec. 84:146-147.

McLaughlin, C.S. M.H. Vaughan, I.M. Campbell, C.M. Wei, M.E. Stafford, and B.S. Hansen. 1977. Inhibition of protein synthesis by trichothecenes, p. 261–284. *In* J. V. Rodricks, C.W. Hesseltine, and M.A. Mehlman (ed.), Mycotoxins in human and animal health. Pathotox Publications, Park Forest South, Ill.

Mirocha, C.J., J. Harrison, A.A. Nichols, and M. McClintock. 1968. Detection of fungal estrogen (F-2) in hay associated with infertility in dairy cattle. Appl. Microbiol. 16:797-798.

Mirocha, C.J., S.V. Pathre, and C.M. Christensen. 1976. Zearalenone. pp. 345-364. In: J.V. Rodricks, C.W. Hesseltine and M.A. Mehlman. (Eds.) "Mycotoxins in Human and Animal Health". Pathotox. Publ., Park Forest, IL.

Mirocha, C.J., B. Schauerhamer, and S.V. Pathre. 1974. Isolation, detection and quantitation of zearalenone in maize and barley. J. Assoc. Off. Anal. Chem. 57:1104-1110.

Nibbelink, S.K. 1986. Aflatoxicosis in food animals: A clinical review. Iowa State Univ. Vet. 48:28-31.

Niyo, K. A., J. L. Richard, Y. Niyo, and L. H. Tiffany. 1988a. Effects of T-2 mycotoxin ingestion on phagocytosis of *Aspergillus fumigatus* conidia by rabbit alveolar macrophages and on hematologic, serum biochemical, and pathologic changes in rabbits. Am J Vet Res 49:1766–1773.

Niyo, K.A., J.L. Richard, Y. Niyo, and L.H. Tiffany. 1988b. Pathologic, hematologic, serologic, and mycologic changes in rabbits given T-2 mycotoxin orally and exposed to aerosols of *Aspergillus fumigatus* conidia. Am J Vet Res 49:2151–2160.

NTP (National Toxicology Program). 1999. Toxicology and carcinogenesis studies on fumonisin B1 in F344/N rats and B6CF1 mice (feed studies). *Technical Report Series, n 496*. NIH Publication No. 99-3955. U.S. Department of Health and Human Services, National Institutes of Health Research Triangle Park, NC.

Osweiler, G.D., M.E. Kehrli, J.R. Stabel, J.R. Thurston, P.F. Ross, and T.M. Wilson. 1993. Effects of fumonisin-contaminated corn screenings on growth and health of feeder calves. J. Anim. Sci. 71:459-466.

Patterson, D.S.P., and P.H. Anderson. 1982. Recent aflatoxin feeding experiments in cattle. Vet. Rec. 110:60-61.

Petrie, L., J. Robb, and A.F. Stewart. 1977. The identification of T-2 toxin and its association with a hemorrhagic syndrome in cattle. Vet. Rec. 101:326-326.

Pier, A.C. 1992. Major biological consequences of aflatoxicosis in animal production. J. Anim. Sci. 70:3964-3970.

Pier A.C., J.L. Richard, and S.J. Cysewski. 1980. The implication of mycotoxins in animal disease. J. Am. Vet. Med. Assoc. 176:719-722.

Puntenney, S.B., Y. Wang, and N.E. Forsberg. 2003. Mycotic infections in livestock: Recent insights and studies on etiology, diagnostics and prevention of Hemorrhagic Bowel Syndrome, In: Southwest Nutrition & Management Conference, Pheonix, University of Arizona, Department of Animal Science, Tuscon, pp. 49-63.

Reeves, E.P., C.G.M. Messina, S. Doyle, and K. Kavanagh. 2004. Correlation between gliotoxin production and virulence of *Aspergillus fumigatus* in *Galleria mellonella.*

Mycopathologia 158:73-79.
Rheeder, J.P., S.F.O. Marassas, P.G. Thiel, E.W. Sydenham, G.S. Spephard, and D.J. VanSchalkwyk. 1992. *Fusarium moniliforme* and fumonisins in corn in relation to human esophageal cancer in Transkei. Phytopathologh 82:353-357.
Roine, K., E.L. Korpinen, and K. Kallela. 1971. Mycotoxicosis as a probable cause of infertility in dairy cows. Nord. Vet. Med. 23:628-633.
Russell, L., D.F. Cox, G. Larsen, K. Bodwell, and C.E Nelson. 1991. Incidence of molds and mycotoxins in commercial animal feed mills in seven Midwestern states, 1988-89. J. Anim. Sci. 69:5-12.
Schiefer, H.B. 1990. Mycotoxicosis of domestic animals and their diagnosis. Can. J. Physiol. Pharmacol. 68:987-990.
Scott, P.M., T. Delgado, D.B. Prelusky, H.L. Trenholm, and J.D. Miller. 1994. Determination of fumonisin in milk. J. Environ. Sci. Health. B29:989-998.
Seglar, B. 1997. Case studies that implicate silage mycotoxins as the cause of dairy herd problems. pp. 242-254. In: "Silage: Field to Feedbunk". NRAES-99, Northeast Regional Agricultural Engineering Service, Ithaca, NY.
Shadmi, A., R. Volcani, and T.A. Nobel. 1974. The pathogenic effect on animals fed mouldy hay or given its etheric fraction. Zentralbl. Veterinaermed. Reihe A. 21:544-552.

Smith, T.K., and E.J. MacDonald. 1991. Effect of fusaric acid on brain regional neurochemistry and vomiting behavior in swine. J. Anim. Sci. 69:2044-2049.
Towers, N.R., J.M. Sprosen, and W. Webber. 1995. Zearalenone metabolites in cycling and non-cycling cows. pp.46-47. In: "Toxinology and Food Safety". Toxinology and Food Safety Research Group, Ruakura Research Centre, Hamilton, New Zealand.
Trenholm, H.L., D.B. Prelusky, J.C. Young, and J.D. Miller. 1988. "Reducing Mycotoxins in Animal Feeds, Publication 1827E, Cat. No. A63-1827/1988E, Agriculture Canada, Ottawa.
Van Egmond, H.P. 1989. Aflatoxin M1: occurrence, toxicity, regulation. pp 11-55. In: Van Egmond, (Ed.) "Mycotoxins in Dairy Products". Elsevier Sci. Pub. Co., Ltd. New York.
Wannemacher, R.W., Jr., D.L. Brunner, and H.A. Neufeld. 1991. Toxicity of trichothecenes and other related mycotoxins in laboratory animals. pp. 499-552. In: J.E. Smith and R.S. Henderson (Eds.), "Mycotoxins and Animal Foods." CRC Press, Inc., Boca Raton, FL.
Weaver, G.A., H.J. Kurtz, J.C. Behrens, T.S. Robison, B.E. Seguin, F.Y. Bates, and C.J. Mirocha 1986a. Effect of zearalenone on the fertility of virgin dairy heifers. Am. J. Vet. Res. 47:1395-1397.
Weaver, G.A., H.J. Kurtz, J.C. Behrens, T.S. Robison, B.E. Seguin, F.Y. Bates, and C.J. Mirocha. 1986b. Effect of zearalenone on dairy cows. Am. J. Vet. Res. 47:1826-1828.
Weaver, G.A., H. J. Kurtz, C.J. Mirocha, F.Y. Bates, J.C. Behrens, T. S. Robison, and S. P. Swanson. 1980. The failure of T-2 mycotoxin to produce hemorrhaging in dairy cattle. Can. Vet. J. 21:210-213.

Whitlow, L.W., and W.M. Hagler, Jr. 2004. Mycotoxins in feeds. Feedstuffs 76 (No. 38):66-76.

Whitlow, L.W., W.M. Hagler, Jr., and B.A. Hopkins. 1998. Mycotoxin occurrence in farmer submitted samples of North Carolina feedstuffs: 1989-1997. J. Dairy Sci. 81(Abstr.):1189.

Whitlow, L.W., R.L. Nebel, and W.M. Hagler, Jr. 1994. The association of deoxynivalenol in grain with milk production loss in dairy cows. Pp. 131-139. In: G.C. Llewellyn, W. V. Dashek and C. E. O=Rear. (Eds.) "Biodeterioration Research 4". Plenum Press, New York.

Whittaker, T.B., J.W. Dickens, and F.G. Giesbrecht. 1991. Testing animal feedstuffs for mycotoxins: sampling, subsampling, and analysis. pp. 153-164. In: J.E. Smith and R.S. Henderson (Eds.), "Mycotoxins and Animal Foods". CRC Press, Boca Raton.

Wood, G.E., and M.W. Trucksess. 1998. Regulatory control programs for mycotoxin-contaminated food. pp. 459-451. In: K.K. Sinha and D. Bhatnagar (Eds.) "Mycotoxins in Agriculture and Food Safety". Markel Dekker, Inc., New York.

Made in the USA
Las Vegas, NV
29 January 2021

16753030R00102